Connie W. Bales is Associate Director of the Sarah W. Stedman Center for Nutritional Studies, Associate Professor of Medicine, and Senior Fellow at the Center for the Study of Aging and Human Development at Duke University Medical Center. She holds a doctorate in Nutrition Science and is also a Registered Dietician.

Marc K. Drezner is a Professor of Medicine and Chief of the Endocrinology, Metabolism and Nutrition Division, as well as Director of the Sarah W. Stedman Center for Nutritional Studies at Duke University Medical Center. He also serves as Editor in Chief of the prestigious *Journal of Bone and Mineral Research*.

Kimberly P. Hoben is a Registered Dietician with a master's degree in public health who conducts research, counsels patients, and teaches nutrition at the Stedman Center.

Dietary Approaches to Healthy Living
from
The Sarah W. Stedman Center
for Nutritional Studies at
Duke University Medical Center

EATING WELL, LIVING WELL
with
OSTEOPOROSIS

Marc K. Drezner, M.D.
Kimberly P. Hoben, R.D., M.P.H., L.D.N.

Connie W. Bales, PH.D., R.D.
Series Editor

with Linda J. Lumsden, PH.D., M.A.

VIKING

VIKING
Published by the Penguin Group
Penguin Books USA Inc., 375 Hudson Street,
New York, New York 10014, U.S.A.
Penguin Books Ltd, 27 Wrights Lane,
London W8 5TZ, England
Penguin Books Australia Ltd, Ringwood,
Victoria, Australia
Penguin Books Canada Ltd, 10 Alcorn Avenue,
Toronto, Ontario, Canada M4V 3B2
Penguin Books (N.Z.) Ltd, 182–190 Wairau Road,
Auckland 10, New Zealand

Penguin Books Ltd, Registered Offices:
Harmondsworth, Middlesex, England

First published in 1996 by Viking Penguin,
a division of Penguin Books USA Inc.

10 9 8 7 6 5 4 3 2 1

Publisher's Note
The ideas, procedures, and suggestions contained in this book are not
intended as a substitute for consulting with your physician. All matters
regarding your health require medical supervision.

Library of Congress Cataloging in Publication Data

Marc K. Drezner.
    Eating well, living well with osteoporosis / [Marc K. Drezner,
  Kimberly P. Hoben].
        p. cm.
    "Dietary approaches to healthy living from the Duke University
  Medical Center written by the staff of the Sarah W. Stedman Center
  for Nutritional Studies."
    Includes resource references and index.
    ISBN 0-670-86659-8
    1. Osteoporosis—Diet therapy.   I. Drezner, Marc K.   II. Hoben,
  Kimberly P.   III. Duke University.   Sarah W. Stedman Center for
  Nutritional Studies.   IV. Title.
  RC931.O73S86   1996
  616.7′16—dc20   95–48764

This book is printed on acid-free paper.

Printed in the United States of America
Set in Minion

Contents

Foreword

Good nutrition is the cornerstone of good health. At the Sarah W. Stedman Center for Nutritional Studies we are committed to the idea that optimum health care includes comprehensive nutritional care. At the Stedman Center, the results of research studies on nutrition and disease are routinely incorporated into the medical/health-care plans of our patients.

The purpose of the *Eating Well, Living Well* book series is to share the expert knowledge of the medical doctors and nutritionists who work within the Duke Medical Center community at the level of nutritional therapy and lifestyle intervention. Education is the key to the prevention and treatment of many common diseases. Yet much of the information available today about nutrition and diet is incomplete and/or inaccurate. We hope that the *Eating Well, Living Well* series will begin to resolve some of the controversies associated with present-day diets.

Many popularly promoted diets are not founded on sound nutritional principles and common sense.

Such diets are difficult for most people to follow, usually because there is no consideration given to those with special health concerns. That is why in each book we include sections on selecting the right foods in a variety of settings, including grocery stores, restaurants, and recreational events. Another problem with catchall and fad diets is that there are often no special allowances made for individual differences in activity, age, or lifestyle.

The *Eating Well, Living Well* book series addresses these issues directly. We have asked experts from specific fields of clinical research and practice to write about disease prevention by nutritional means, with specific emphasis on individual differences and exceptions to the rules. Each book is uniquely tailored for each disease. This one explores the latest nutritional aspects of osteoporosis, a serious bone disease that can affect adult men and women of all ages.

Sarah White Stedman
September 1995

Chapter One

What Is Osteoporosis?

If you're like most people, you hope that when you retire you can travel to new places, play with your grandchildren, pursue leisure activities such as gardening, and/or participate in recreational sports such as golf or tennis.

But imagine that your bones are brittle. So brittle that you cannot pick up a bag of groceries, let alone lift your grandchild in the air without worry. Imagine that the threat of breaking a bone doesn't just limit your travel plans, it makes even turning over in bed feel risky.

This scenario is an unfortunate reality for some of the 25 million Americans—80 percent of them women—who suffer from osteoporosis.

Osteoporosis is a chronic degenerative bone disease in which the body loses excessive amounts of bone; the diminished bone leaves the skeleton weak, brittle, and susceptible to fractures, especially in the spine, hip, and wrists. Osteoporosis, which literally means "porous bones," is often called a silent disease, because it progresses without symptoms until a fracture causing pain occurs. There are several different types of osteoporosis, some of which are caused by other medical factors.

The most common forms of osteoporosis are **postmenopausal** and **senile osteoporosis.** Postmenopausal osteoporosis most often affects women between 50 and 65 years of age; senile osteoporosis develops in men and women 65 years of age or older. The separation of these two forms of the disease is somewhat arbitrary. Both occur to differing degrees as a natural consequence of aging.

In contrast, **steroid-induced osteoporosis,** another common form of the disease, is a complication that often occurs in patients treated long-term with corticosteroid drugs such as prednisone.

The most common visible sign of osteoporosis is the so-called dowager's hump, the hunched upper back sometimes seen in elderly women. This is the result of multiple fractures of the spinal vertebrae (backbones), which frequently collapse when they fracture. But even a collapsed vertebra may be painless or cause so little pain that a woman is unaware of the problem and may not think of seeking medical help until she notices her hunched posture or a measurable reduction in height.

Since postmenopausal osteoporosis is by far the most common form of the disease, it is a major women's health problem, and the most common metabolic bone disease in the developed world. A woman's risk of experiencing a hip fracture during her lifetime, more likely when she has "porous bones," is equal to her combined risk of developing breast, uterine, and ovarian cancer.

A staggering one out of two American women over the age of 65 will experience fractures because of the disease. Men are not immune, either: one out of five men 65 years of age or older will also suffer fractures due to osteoporosis.

This disabling disease also takes a psychological toll.

As a person deals with varying levels of chronic pain and physical disfigurement, self-esteem can plummet and stress levels can rise. It becomes harder and harder to perform "normal" daily activities, join in recreational pursuits, cook, or do simple household chores. With depression can come apathy, loss of appetite, sleep disorders, and strained relationships with friends and family.

Triad of Treatment

Fortunately, the common forms of osteoporosis are largely preventable and/or treatable. We propose a three-pronged strategy involving proper nutrition, exercise, and drug therapy. This may prevent, delay, or alleviate postmenopausal, senile, and steroid-induced osteoporosis. Nutrition plays a fundamental role in this triad, largely because it is the safest and least complicated way to prevent and treat osteoporosis. Without optimal nutrition, the other two components of the triad would be severely compromised.

This book will explain osteoporosis to you and tell you how you can determine if you are at risk for the diseases. It will explain how you can use the triad of treatment to avoid this disease or mitigate its effects. Most important, it will emphasize the role nutrition can play in preventing or delaying the symptoms of osteoporosis, and the importance of calcium in any and all treatment programs.

You will learn how to shop for foods high in calcium and prepare calcium-rich meals—assisted by high-calcium recipes created by nutritionists at the Stedman Center and featured in chapter nine. Maintaining a high calcium intake when eating away from home can be a real challenge. This is addressed in chapter ten.

Though the focus of this book is clearly on nutrition, we will also discuss the role of exercise and drug therapy in treating and/or preventing osteoporosis, since they can all work together for optimal bone health. Before discussing how to improve bone health, let's take a look at bones and the essential roles they play in the body.

The Importance of Bones

The 206 bones in the skeletal system form the framework for the human body. They determine our physical shape, protect our organs, store calcium and other minerals for the rest of the body, provide leverage, and enable us to move. Bones work in conjunction with ligaments, which connect them at the joints, and muscles, which attach to bones via tendons.

If we think about them at all, we usually picture bones as lifeless and hard. Every bone, however, is a complex, living tissue made of proteins and minerals, including calcium.

Our bones are composed of two kinds of tissue. **Cortical bone** makes up the dense, hard shell in the outer layer of most bones. In contrast, **trabecular bone** is spongier and porous. It forms the inner layer of bone that surrounds the bone marrow, which is composed of blood vessels, fat cells, and blood-forming cells. An adult skeleton contains about 80 percent cortical bone and 20 percent trabecular bone. Long, straight bones such as the femur consist primarily of cortical bone; more flexible bones such as ribs and vertebrae are composed mainly of trabecular bone. It is important to know the two types of bone tissue and where they are located, because they are affected differently during bone loss.

Bones constantly change throughout our lives. As old bone is resorbed (or broken down) to repair microfractures (tiny injuries to bone that happen in the course of daily living and do not require medical attention) and/or to provide calcium to the circulation, new bone replaces

Normal Bone Remodeling

1. Resting Phase

A resting bone surface covered by lining cells shows no evidence of remodeling.

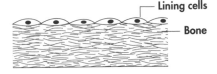

2. Resorption

During resorption, multi-nucleated giant cells called osteoclasts are attracted to the bone surface and excavate the bone, dissolving the mineral and matrix and creating cavities, or Howship's lacunae.

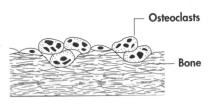

3. Reversal

With the completion of resorption, the osteoclasts disappear and leave the large cavities, which are invaded by small cells with single nuclei.

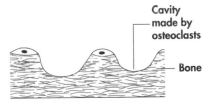

4. Formation (Repair)

A team of bone-forming cells called osteoblasts deposit new, unmineralized bone in the cavities and guide the ultimate calcification of the bone.

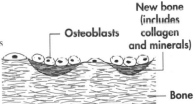

5. Completed Repair

At the completion of bone formation, osteoblasts have been replaced by flattened lining cells, and the bone surface has been completely restored.

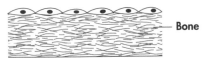

it. This process of resorbing and then replacing bone is called **bone remodeling.**

Bone Remodeling

The bone-remodeling process keeps bones healthy and strong. Two kinds of cells are involved in remodeling:

Osteoclasts resorb existing bone by dissolving tiny areas of bone tissue so that the calcium it contains can be moved into the bloodstream. Bone resorption leaves behind tiny cavities (**Howship's lacunae**) in the bone.

Osteoblasts fill these cavities with a substance primarily made up of a protein called **collagen.** Within two weeks, the filling material begins to harden or mineralize. In this process, calcium and phosphate are embedded in the bone in the form of calcium-phosphate crystals.

The critical factor for healthy bones is a high bone mass, the primary determinant for which is **bone density.** And the essential mineral nutrient calcium is crucial in determining bone density. When the body builds more bone than it destroys, bone density and bone mass increase; when the body destroys more bone than it builds, bone density and bone mass decrease.

Bone density rises and falls throughout our lives depending upon several factors. The most important factors are age and, in women, the estrogen deficiency associated with menopause.

How Age Affects Bone Mass

Bone growth in utero and during childhood is extremely rapid. During these periods of development and growth, bone-building cells rapidly outpace bone-destroying cells to build longer and more dense bones.

With the onset of puberty and during the teenage years, the production of estrogen by the ovaries in girls, and testosterone by the testes in boys, help bones grow stronger. When a child stops growing, bone mass continues to increase in width because the body continues to make much more bone than it destroys until the body achieves peak bone mass, sometime between the ages of 20 and 30 years.

It is evident that these early years of life provide a unique opportunity to build up bone strength. The body begins to lose bone mass after reaching this watershed point. *The level of bone density at the time of peak bone mass is a crucial determining factor for having healthy bones for the rest of your life.*

As the time of peak bone mass passes, the body becomes progressively less efficient at metabolizing calcium. As a consequence, bone resorption begins to outpace bone formation. Most people lose 0.3 to 0.5 percent of bone mass annually after achieving peak mass. Even more alarming for women is that loss of bone mass rises geometrically after the menopause.

Menopause and Reduced Estrogen

With the onset of menopause (usually around 50 years of age), women become especially vulnerable to osteoporosis because they are producing less estrogen. Decreased estrogen production triggers a series of events that result in increased bone resorption. Research studies indicate that estrogen diminishes osteoclast activity (and thus helps reduce the rate of bone resorption) by direct interaction with the cell. Estrogen also naturally suppresses the production of bone-resorbing **cytokines,** or protein mediators. Thus, reducing estrogen increases the rate of bone resorption because of unregulated osteoclast and cytokine activity.

In the 10 years following menopause or surgical removal of the ovaries, estrogen deficiency generally results in a minimum loss of 10 percent of cortical-bone mass and another 25 percent of trabecular-bone mass. Eventually, approximately 10 years after the menopause, the rate of bone loss slows considerably—to about 1 percent a year.

For these reasons, a woman can expect to lose 35 percent of cortical bone and 50 percent of trabecular bone over her lifetime. It is not surprising that bone fractures usually begin to occur about 10 to 15 years following menopause, because that's when the rate of bone loss has peaked.

In contrast, men begin to lose bone mass typically about 10 years later than women and at a slower, steadier rate of about 1 percent a year. As a consequence, men usually undergo only about two-thirds of the bone loss that women experience in a lifetime. A man may still encounter bone loss leading to fractures if his peak bone mass was low and/or if he lives to an advanced age.

Who Is at Risk?

Age and gender are the most significant factors in determining who will get osteoporosis: everyone's bones become weaker and less dense as they age, but older women are at the greatest risk. Other factors also may predispose a person to the disease. Some of the most common factors include:

Body size
Petite women with small frames are at increased risk of developing osteoporosis. Many studies have correlated low measurements of body fat to increased rates of vertebral and hip fractures. Men with small frames are also at a greater risk for osteoporosis.

Race

Several epidemiological investigations reveal that Caucasian and Asian women are at the greatest risk of developing osteoporosis. Hispanic and African-American women are also at risk.

Estrogen deficiency

Early menopause (before age 45), surgical removal of the ovaries, and long-term transient amenorrhea (abnormal absence of menstruation) also predispose women to osteoporosis unless they receive estrogen-replacement therapy.

Calcium deficiency and related dietary factors

When you don't take in enough calcium to meet the needs of your body, your body compensates by removing calcium from bones—calcium that is needed to rebuild bone and keep bones strong. Thus, an adequate intake of calcium is essential for optimum bone health. Other dietary factors common in Western diets may reduce calcium balance and increase the risk of osteoporosis.

Medications

Corticosteroids such as Prednisone are synthetically created hormones used as anti-inflammatory drugs to treat a number of diseases, including rheumatoid arthritis, asthma, lupus erythematosus, Crohn's disease, ulcerative colitis, and multiple sclerosis. Steroids are also prescribed for cancer patients undergoing chemotherapy, and for recipients of organ transplants. In addition to their powerful anti-inflammatory benefits, these drugs possess a number of negative side effects. They interfere with bone remodeling, causing rapid bone loss at the inception of therapy and a slower rate of loss during the long-term treatment course. Anyone receiving long-term steroid therapy should take calcium supplements (see chapter four) and be aware of other risk factors for osteoporosis. In addition to corticosteroids, other prescription drugs that can adversely affect bone include:

- aluminum-containing antacids
- cholestyramine
- cyclosporine A
- gonadotropin-releasing hormone analogues
- heparin
- methotrexate
- phenytoin and barbiturate anticonvulsants
- thyroid hormones

Coexistent disease

Osteoporosis can be a complication of several medical conditions, including hyperthyroidism, removal of the small colon, Type I diabetes mellitus, anorexia nervosa, and prolonged parenteral nutrition. Hospitalized patients and others who are bedridden for prolonged periods of time also experience rapid bone loss, which may result in osteoporosis.

Smoking and drinking

Cigarettes and excessive alcohol have been associated with an increase in bone loss and consequent development of osteoporosis. Both are toxic to bone-building cells.

Lack of exercise

Weight-bearing exercises help strengthen bones. Walking, jogging, and playing tennis are examples of weight-bearing exercises that work the muscles against gravity. Rapid bone loss occurs in anyone who becomes immobilized because of any accident or illness and cannot participate in regular weight-bearing exercise. It follows that sedentary people are at greater risk for osteoporosis.

Heredity

Genetic factors may play a role in determining who gets osteoporosis. Studies show that women whose mothers suffered vertebral fractures, suggesting they suffered from osteoporosis, also seem to have inherited lower bone mass.

Detecting Osteoporosis

Until recently, the silent nature of osteoporosis during its development phase made its detection difficult. Recent technological advances have provided physicians with new diagnostic tests that permit accurate and precise detection of decreased bone mass well before the fracture threshold is reached—particularly valuable since osteoporosis gives no warning of its presence until it is so far advanced that debilitating fractures occur.

Conventional X-rays can detect osteoporosis only after 25 to 30 percent of bone is lost. In contrast, several tests have been developed that are dedicated to measuring bone density and can detect bone loss much earlier. These tests are for the most part noninvasive and painless.

The most common bone-density tests project radiation energy of multiple wavelengths through a bone; the tests measure the fraction of the energy passing through. The more dense the bone, measured in terms of bone-calcium content, the smaller the amount of radiation that will pass through it.

Testing is recommended:

- for all women with reduced estrogen who are at risk (including those at the menopause) to make decisions about hormone-replacement therapy.
- in men and women with vertebral abnormalities or

X-ray evidence suggesting bone loss to confirm the presence of spinal osteoporosis.
- in patients receiving long-term corticosteroid therapy to identify low bone mass.
- to assess the effects of long-term therapy for osteoporosis.

The most accurate and precise of the bone-measurement techniques developed over the past two decades is **dual-energy X-ray absorptiometry (DXA).** This state-of-the-art test permits assessment of bone mass in all three primary potential fracture sites—hip, spinal vertebrae, and wrists—in less than 20 minutes. The results are analyzed by computer, which allows calculation of the bone density and plotting of the data on a scale specific to sex, age, and race. Your readings can be compared with those of a person at peak bone mass. This can help identify whether you are at risk for osteoporosis long before a fracture occurs. In addition, these measurements can provide a guide for treatment strategies before the patient has any symptoms of disease.

DXA is not necessary for everyone. You and your doctor should decide whether you should have this test after weighing factors that affect your risk, such as heredity, medical history, drug therapy, lifestyle, and diet. Radiation exposure is minimal, and the procedure is painless, since it involves only lying quietly in a comfortable position.

Quantitative computed tomography (CT scan) is also used to evaluate bone mass. For this measurement, you lie on your back in a large cylindrical tube while the machine scans your skeleton for about 20 minutes. The three-dimensional images the CT scan produces allow your doctor to distinguish between cortical and trabecular bone. However, experts disagree on the test's accuracy,

CT scans are expensive, and they emit far more radiation than DXA.

Physicians may also ask for blood and urine samples when testing for osteoporosis because these fluids contain materials that can help determine how the body's metabolism is functioning. Such tests help your doctor evaluate your rate of bone loss.

The Next Step

If you are diagnosed with osteoporosis or significantly low bone density, the triad of treatment for osteoporosis—nutrition, exercise, and drug therapy—becomes an important concern for you.

Almost all people can prevent or decrease the severity of the disease if they commit themselves to the first two legs (nutrition and exercise) of the triad throughout their lifetime. You can lessen risk of osteoporosis by consistently eating well, especially by taking in sufficient calcium. You can help ensure that your bones stay healthy and strong by getting weight-bearing exercise. If you are at risk for osteoporosis, incorporating calcium and exercise into your lifestyle can significantly reduce that risk. Even if you have osteoporosis, good nutrition that concentrates on a calcium-rich diet along with a weight-bearing exercise program can delay or mitigate symptoms.

Good nutrition and exercise may make drug therapy, the third leg of the triad, unnecessary for many people. Even people who undergo drug therapy, however, whether they have osteoporosis or are at risk of the disease, need a calcium-rich diet and a good exercise program to ward off fractures and stay on their feet. The triad strategy works best when all three factors work together.

Chapter Two

The Triad of Treatment for Osteoporosis

Although we will focus on nutrition, which is the foundation of the triad of treatment for osteoporosis, exercise and drug therapy are also important components of any program to combat the disease. One big advantage of exercise as a strategy for countering osteoporosis is that it harbors none of the potentially harmful side effects associated with all forms of hormonal and drug treatments for the disease. Another bonus is that exercise contributes to your overall health: improving cardiovascular fitness, toning muscle, preventing obesity, lowering your risk of disease, and extending life expectancy.

Exercise as Prevention

Once a person has reached peak bone mass, **weight-bearing exercise** is the only *known* way to increase bone density without therapeutic intervention. Weight-bearing exercises are those that work the muscles against gravity or through muscular contraction. Exercises that combine movement, pull, and stress on the long bones of the body do the most for bone health. Second to getting adequate dietary calcium, pursuing a regular program of exercise is one of the easiest and most effective ways for young people to prevent osteoporosis. In addition, we will see that exercise can also help ease pain and delay fractures in individuals who already have osteoporosis.

As mentioned in chapter one, a sedentary lifestyle can, in fact, cause an increase in bone loss. The amount of bone tissue actually decreases when people stop getting exercise because of an accident or illness that puts them off their feet. Even otherwise healthy people lose bone if they stop doing weight bearing exercise. Astronauts lose bone when they are weightless during prolonged flights in space. In contrast, female marathon runners with normal menstrual periods have been found to have greater bone mass than inactive women the same age. The more active the muscle that covers bone, the denser the bone seems to be.

Some weight-bearing exercises recommended by the National Osteoporosis Foundation to help build bone include:

- alpine skiing
- basketball
- cross-country skiing
- dancing
- ice skating
- jogging
- soccer

- stair climbing
- tennis
- volleyball
- walking
- water aerobics
- weight training

Though not as effective as the activities listed above, training on such exercise equipment as cross-country ski machines and stair machines helps build up bone with less stress on the body than the activities above. Swimming is excellent for toning muscle and offering a cardiovascular workout, but it is not especially helpful in building up bone because it does not work the muscles against gravity. Scientists are unsure about the benefits of bicycling for bone health.

An exercise program for osteoporosis does not have to be expensive or complicated. Walking, for instance, is excellent, because it strengthens the back, leg, and stomach muscles in addition to stimulating bone growth.

The only caveat about exercise for young women is that extremely strenuous and prolonged athletic training can cause amenorrhea, cessation of menstrual periods because of low estrogen levels. Amenorrhea raises the risk of developing osteoporosis. One study of competitive women runners who failed to menstruate revealed they had 28 percent less bone mass than other women of similar age. The cause of this bone loss remains controversial.

Exercise as Therapy

The good news for individuals with osteoporosis is this: research shows that embarking upon a program of regular exercise can help reduce bone loss among people who already have osteoporosis. In one study, subjects engaged in weight-bearing exercises at least three times a week for 30 to 45 minutes over a period of eight months to three years. *The result was a reduction in their rate of bone loss.* Other studies show that age is no barrier to getting good results from an exercise routine. Bone mass actually *increased* by 4 percent among a group of women aged 69 and older who followed a regulated exercise program.

So what are the exercises you can do if you already have symptoms that restrict your physical activities?

There are a number of beneficial activities to choose from, *provided that your physician and physical therapist approve.* Isometric exercises—exercises that contract muscles—can exert force or stress on the spine to aid in stimulating bone growth. Pelvic tilts, isometric head presses, and chest, leg, and arm lifts can be performed in a sitting or prostrate position to strengthen your back, hip, and abdominal muscles safely, as well as to increase flexibility. Such exercises can be crucial if your mobility is highly restricted, which can make you highly susceptible to accelerated bone loss.

Exercise can help reduce your risk of serious and even life-threatening injuries such as hip fractures by making you stronger and more flexible and thus less likely to fall. It also provides a physical outlet for coping with stress that can make it easier to deal with your osteoporosis, as well as other stress in your daily life.

It is imperative to get medical clearance before embarking upon any exercise program—so that you don't put undue stress on your bones and risk an injury. Ask your doctor and physical therapist how to begin an exercise routine. They can recommend exercises that are appropriate for your needs and ability.

Avoiding Falls in Your Home

Preventing falls is especially important for people who have osteoporosis, since they can result in a broken hip or other bones. Here are some tips on how to avoid falls in your home:

- Install sturdy handrails on staircases.
- Put light switches at the top and bottom of staircases.

Avoiding Falls in Your Home *(cont'd.)*

- Mark the first and last steps with bright tape.
- Install grab bars along shower walls and next to toilets.
- Install a shower seat and portable, hand-held shower head in the bathtub so you can sit while showering.
- Provide ample lighting throughout your home, including a bedside light and a night light between your bedroom and bathroom.
- Keep your home free of clutter so you don't trip over items such as long telephone cords.
- Arrange furniture so it does not create obstacles.
- Keep kitchen utensils and other tools within easy reach to avoid climbing on footstools.
- Use a long-handled grasping device to reach faraway items.
- Cover slippery floors with nonskid area rugs or carpet that is firmly anchored to the floor.
- Use nonskid floor wax on linoleum floors.
- Talk to your physician to determine if any medications you take will affect your balance or coordination.
- Limit your alcohol intake, since drinking can impair your balance.

Persons with osteoporosis often need more intensive intervention than can be provided by diet or exercise. These treatments include calcium supplements and calcitonin, biophosphonates, estrogen, or experimental drug therapy. The most widespread—and controversial—of these therapies is estrogen, or **hormone-replacement therapy (HRT).**

Hormone-Replacement Therapy

Women today can expect to live 20 to 30 years after reaching menopause at about age 50. The loss of bone mass is among the most serious of several adverse effects brought on by the loss of estrogen that accompanies menopause. Estrogen loss may also increase women's risk of heart attack and cause a host of unpleasant side effects, including sweating, hot flashes, painful sexual intercourse, painful urination, frequent need to urinate, muscle and joint aches, backache, headache, insomnia, and depression.

Estrogen not only alleviates these symptoms but may dramatically delay the onset of osteoporosis. Estrogen slows the rate of bone loss in postmenopausal women. A Swedish study showed that the risk of hip fractures is decreased by 60 percent in postmenopausal women who take estrogen supplements; similarly, the rate for vertebral crush fractures among these women is 60 to 80 percent of the rate among those who do not take estrogen. Clearly, estrogen is a most effective means to reduce fractures in older women, keeping them on their feet and out of nursing homes.

Such efficacy explains why HRT is considered by many physicians an appropriate regimen for women over the age of 50. Doctors frequently recommend the use of estrogen therapy for at least five to 10 years following menopause or for a woman's lifetime. In fact, recent research indicates that even after vertebral fracture occurs, initiating estrogen therapy protects bone mass and prevents further fractures.

Conjugated equine estrogen, the drug most frequently used in HRT, under the brand name Premarin, is the most prescribed drug in the United States. HRT combines the estrogen with the synthetic female sex hormone progesterone. Treatment involves several different possible regimens. Perhaps the most common requires taking estrogen pills for three weeks followed by progestin pills for about 10 days. Alternatively, some women wear an estrogen patch that transmits a form of estrogen called **estradiol** transdermally, or through the skin. Most experts believe that to maximize its benefits, HRT should begin at the first signs of menopause.

Despite the obvious benefits of HRT, significant controversy surrounds the use of estrogens in post-menopausal women. This powerful therapy, like so many drug regimens, is not entirely benign. The most serious side effect is an apparent association between estrogen and increased rates of uterine and breast cancer. However, research shows that the addition of progestin reduces the risk of uterine cancer, and many doctors believe the kinds and amounts of estrogen used in the United States are not associated with breast cancer. Perhaps more important, the potentially increased risk of breast cancer is overcome by the improved life expectancy that results from protection against heart disease and hip fracture, among other maladies. Nevertheless, women with undiagnosed vaginal bleeding or a history of breast cancer should not undergo HRT.

Some women decline to use estrogen or other sex hormones because of the unanswered questions about other potential negative effects, including:

- benign tumors of the uterus
- bloating
- breast tenderness or enlargement
- cancer of the breast or uterus
- depression
- facial skin spots and darkening
- gallstones
- nausea
- vaginal bleeding
- vaginal yeast infections

- difficulty wearing contact lenses
- dizziness
- venous thrombosis

A couple of alternative drug therapies that help slow bone loss are available to osteoporosis patients, and are especially valuable for women unable or unwilling to undergo HRT. The treatments include the recently approved calcitonin and biophosphonates.

Calcitonin Supplements

Calcitonin, a naturally occurring hormone produced primarily in the thyroid gland, limits the release of calcium from bone into the bloodstream. The calcitonin works directly on the osteoclasts to stop bone breakdown, primarily affecting trabecular bone. This action serves to slow bone loss due to menopause and aging. In addition, several studies indicate that calcitonin relieves the pain of vertebral fractures.

Two major drawbacks to this treatment are its cost, which may exceed several thousand dollars a year, and its inconvenience. Unfortunately, patients cannot take calcitonin in pill form, since the digestive enzymes in the stomach destroy the hormone before it is absorbed in the body. Calcitonin must be administered by injection. Patients may travel to a doctor's office for shots or train themselves to administer an injection one to three times a week, depending on the dose required. To make calcitonin effective, patients must also take 1,000 milligrams of calcium daily, through diet or calcium supplements.

The hormone also has its share of transient side effects, including flushing of the face, frequent urination, nausea, and rashes. And some people develop a resistance to calcitonin, rendering it less effective during long-term treatment.

Biophosphonates

Biophosphonates are another class of drugs used for treating osteoporosis. After extensive investigation, the Food and Drug Administration (FDA) has begun to approve selective representatives of this drug class for treatment of osteoporosis. When administered intermittently, biophosphonates appear to reduce postmenopausal bone loss, particularly in the spine, by inhibiting the bone-resorption process. **Sodium alendronate** is one of the biophosphonates recently approved for use. Studies indicate that after a year to 18 months, it not only slows bone loss but can also increase vertebral bone mass 5 to 7 percent in postmenopausal women. A major drawback of biophosphonates is that they may cause serious gastrointestinal disturbances. And their long-term effects remain unknown, so that their future role in the management of osteoporosis is as yet ill-defined.

Experimental Treatments

Research is under way on a number of experimental drug treatments not yet approved by the FDA that hold promise for people with osteoporosis.

Etidronate, another biophosphonate, is a potent inhibitor of mineralization, but its efficacy remains unproven. Researchers are investigating a **nasal-spray calcitonin**, which would be more convenient to use than injections. The nasal spray has been used effectively to reduce bone loss among younger postmenopausal women and to reduce the number of spinal fractures in elderly osteoporosis patients. Daily injections of a synthetic **human parathyroid hormone (hPTH)** have been shown to increase trabecular bone by 40 to 50 percent in postmenopausal women with osteoporosis when combined with administration of estrogen or androgens for a year. **Sodium-fluoride** treatment involves the daily use of pills containing 40 to 60 milligrams that appear to stimulate osteoblasts and trabecular-bone growth. **Raloxifene** is an experimental drug structurally similar to estrogen that prevents bone loss. Tests in animals without ovaries and postmenopausal women look promising but remain incomplete. The synthetic antiestrogen **tamoxifen,** which has been used to treat breast cancer, has also been shown to diminish bone loss. However, it may entail such severe side effects that its use must be restricted to women with breast cancer. Several additional experimental drugs have been identified that increase new bone formation. These agents, including **IGF-1** and **zeolite A,** stimulate osteoblasts and bone growth. Toxicity trials in humans and evaluation of the effects on fracture rates will determine whether such agents may herald new forms of treatment for osteoporosis.

Fractures among the elderly have also been reduced by the administration of **vitamin-D supplements,** but doses substantially larger than the recommended 800 international units (IU) daily carry significant risk of increased urinary calcium, elevated blood calcium, and, in some cases, enhanced bone resorption. **Calcitriol,** an active metabolite of vitamin D, also reduces bone loss and lessens the risk of vertebral fractures, but may cause problems similar to those encountered with high doses of vitamin D.

Finding Professional Help for Osteoporosis

It is imperative that you get qualified professionals to help you cope with or prevent osteoporosis and to discuss such important issues as the appropriateness of HRT therapy and the seriousness of osteoporosis in general.

Some physicians are more expert in treating osteoporosis than others. If osteoporosis is a serious problem for you that has defied traditional intervention, seek help from an endocrinologist, a rheumatologist, or an orthopedist with subspecialty training in the management of bone diseases.

One underused source of nutritional expertise is a registered dietitian (**R.D.**). An R.D. has earned a bachelor-of-science degree in nutrition and can counsel you on how best to attain a calcium-rich diet. Most states require that registered dietitians be licensed to do nutritional counseling. These professionals identify themselves as "R.D., L.D." (or "L.D.N."). Ask your physician for a referral, or call the referral number for the American Dietetic Association listed in the Resources section of this book. Other valid food authorities are scientists with a doctoral degree in nutrition. These professionals are usually involved in research on nutrition to cure or treat disease, and do not ordinarily practice clinical nutrition. The Stedman Center employs many such professionals, including R.D.'s, L.D.'s, Ph.D.'s, and M.D.'s, who engage in a wide range of nutritional-research projects and clinical programs.

Nutrition at the Foundation of the Triad

Regardless of the drug therapy and exercise regimen employed to fight osteoporosis, however, nutrition remains the fundamental base of the triad of treatment.

Sound nutrition with a diet rich in high calcium sources at its core remains the safest, easiest way to prevent or slow the onset or progression of osteoporosis. Without sufficient calcium in your diet, you may severely limit the successful prevention or treatment of osteoporosis. Two principles govern the management of osteoporosis: (1) you can prevent or retard the onset of osteoporosis by eating enough calcium throughout your life; and (2) treatment of osteoporosis in women after menopause is more efficient when they also receive high amounts of calcium.

Research from around the world shows that the surest way to accrue sufficient bone and stymie bone loss is to maintain high calcium levels throughout life. The best strategy for avoiding osteoporosis is early prevention. If you already have symptoms of the condition or know you are at high risk of developing osteoporotic fractures, don't panic. It's never too late to start a program to build back bone mass.

If you don't yet have symptoms, you are ahead of the game. You can tailor your nutrition and lifestyle to reduce significantly the chances that you will join the 25 million Americans whose quality of life has been robbed by the silent thief. You can also impress upon your daughters or granddaughters the importance and relative ease of early prevention. Pass along to them the principles of good nutrition, to which you will be introduced in chapter three.

Bone Building for Kids

Let your children or grandchildren know there are lots of things they can do to build strong bones. Children build the skeleton that must support them for the rest of their lives. However, studies show that a third of children under age five get only about 75 percent of the recommended daily intake of calcium.

At the Stedman Center, we recommend that children aged 10 years or younger ingest 800 to 1,200 milligrams of calcium a day (see chapter four). Older children and teens need 1,200 to 1,500 milligrams a day. That means consuming as much as five glasses of milk or the equivalent in calcium a day.

Girls especially need to get plenty of calcium when they start menstruating. Teenagers often drink soda instead of milk at a time when they need milk more than ever. Teenage girls are vulnerable to cultural pressures that encourage them to diet, which discourages them from getting enough nutrients through normal diets. Studies show that only one in four American teens gets enough calcium on a daily basis. Impress upon the teenage girls in your life the importance of building a strong skeleton now. Introduce them to nonfat dairy products and calcium-fortified fruit juices to expand their options for adding calcium to their diet.

Encourage teens—and even younger children—to learn how to read food labels. Discourage them from using alcohol, tobacco, or caffeine, all of which rob calcium from bone.

Children are also building bones when they play—as long as their day includes plenty of weight-bearing exercise, such as running, jumping rope, or playing basketball. Countering osteoporosis is just one more reason children should be encouraged to lead an active life. Here are some easy ways children can be more active:

- Walk to school or other places instead of riding in a car.
- Join a sports team or take a karate or gymnastics class.
- Walk up stairs instead of taking an elevator.
- Turn off the television and go outside to play.

Chapter Three

Nutrition for Overall Good Health and Bone Health

The best way to make sure you are getting enough bone-building calcium is to eat a healthy, balanced diet. Such a diet features a variety of foods, including several servings of calcium-rich foods each day. It offers lots of benefits besides strong bones. Eating well improves your entire physical and emotional well-being and reduces your risk of cancer, heart disease, diabetes, and obesity.

Beliefs about what constitutes a balanced diet have evolved over the years as researchers have learned more about the deleterious effects of excessive amounts of fats (especially saturated fats), alcohol, calories, sugar, and salt, and the benefits of grains, fruits, vegetables, lean meats and other proteins, and low-fat dairy products.

The Stedman Center advises that you follow the general nutritional guidelines illustrated by the Food Guide Pyramid, created in 1992 by the U.S. Department of Agriculture and the U.S. Department of Health and Human Services. The pyramid replaces the Basic Four Food Groups created by Harvard University's Department of Nutrition in the early 1950s and adopted by the Department of Agriculture in 1957. The new Food Guide Pyramid describes a diet lower in saturated fat and includes many more fruits, vegetables, and grains than the old Basic Four recommendations most of us grew up with.

Using the Food Guide Pyramid

The new pyramid makes it easy to visualize how grains, rice, and pasta form the foundation of a healthy diet. It divides foods into six groups. Just as the bottom of the pyramid forms its largest part, so grains, rice, and pasta form the foundation of your daily diet (see page 30). You should eat at least six servings a day from this group. A serving equals one slice of bread, an ounce of cereal, or ½ cup of cooked pasta or rice.

The second tier of the pyramid contains vegetables and fruits. You should eat at least three servings of vegetables a day. A serving equals a cup of raw leafy vegetables, ¾ cup of vegetable juice, or ½ cup of cooked vegetables. You should also eat at least two fruits a day. One serving equals one medium raw fruit, three-quarters cup of fruit juice, or one-half cup of cooked, canned fruit.

On the third tier are the dairy group and the protein group. At the very least, you should get two or three servings from the dairy group daily. One serving from the dairy group equals a cup of milk or yogurt or 1½ ounces of cheese. You should also get at least two to three servings from the protein group. One serving of protein equals two to three ounces of cooked lean meat, fish, or poultry; two eggs; or one cup of cooked beans.

Butter, sour cream, oil, shortening, sugar, and margarine are found primarily in the pyramid's sixth food group, at the narrow tip of the pyramid. These products should be used sparingly, because they provide fat but virtually no other nutrients.

The idea behind the pyramid is that anyone who eats some foods from the first five groups every day will receive adequate amounts of the more than 50 nutrients identified as essential to human health. Bread, rice, pasta, and grains supply us with carbohydrates, iron, and many of the B vitamins, such as thiamin and niacin. Fruits and vegetables are our major sources of vitamins A and C, as well as fiber, which aids digestion. Meat and its substitutes are major sources of protein, B vitamins, and minerals such as zinc and iron. Dairy products supply protein and thiamin but, most important, 76 percent of our calcium.

When you're at risk for osteoporosis and other nutrient-dependent diseases, you will probably have to modify the Food Guide Pyramid guidelines. The recommendation of two to three daily servings of dairy products is too modest. The Stedman Center recommendation for those at risk for osteoporosis is four to five daily servings of low-fat dairy products to increase the daily intake of the bone-building mineral calcium.

Calcium Versus Fat

Although dairy is the champion of calcium sources, many dairy products also are high in fat. This poses a challenge for people who want to get lots of calcium from dairy foods but also want to limit their fat intake, especially saturated fat. Some cheeses are loaded with saturated fat.

Fortunately, you can eat dairy products without taking in too much fat by choosing from among the myriad low-fat and nonfat dairy products that have appeared on dairy shelves in recent years. These products are also low in cholesterol or cholesterol-free, and they contain fewer calories than regular dairy products.

Reducing the amount of fat in dairy products does not reduce the amount of calcium they contain; in fact, skim milk contains slightly more calcium than whole milk. The process removes only the fat portion of the milk.

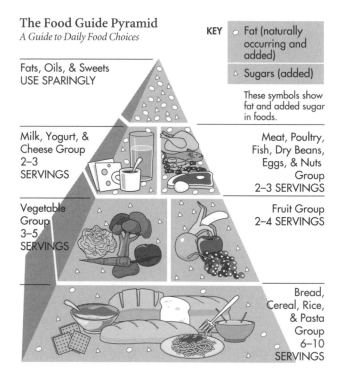

The Food Guide Pyramid
A Guide to Daily Food Choices

KEY
○ Fat (naturally occurring and added)
△ Sugars (added)

These symbols show fat and added sugar in foods.

Fats, Oils, & Sweets
USE SPARINGLY

Milk, Yogurt, & Cheese Group
2–3 SERVINGS

Meat, Poultry, Fish, Dry Beans, Eggs, & Nuts Group
2–3 SERVINGS

Vegetable Group
3–5 SERVINGS

Fruit Group
2–4 SERVINGS

Bread, Cereal, Rice, & Pasta Group
6–10 SERVINGS

Nutrition and Aging

The older you get, the greater your need for calcium and general good nutrition. Many factors combine to enhance the likelihood of bone loss in older people. For one thing, as their metabolic rates decline, the elderly need fewer calories to maintain ideal body weight, so they take in proportionately less calcium no matter how well balanced their diet. A 21-year-old woman may consume 2,900 calories daily, whereas a 75-year-old woman may need only 1,600 calories daily to maintain her weight. Her intake of calcium with this reduction will decrease unless her diet is specially designed.

It's also important to pay attention to your vitamin-D levels. Vitamin D is responsible for calcium absorption. Poorer kidney function and less exposure to vitamin-D-producing sunlight also mean decreased calcium absorption.

Poverty and/or prolonged illness further affect bone health in many elderly people. The one-fifth of the elderly population who live below the poverty level have trouble affording food to meet basic nutritional needs. Nearly a third of some 28 million Americans aged 65 and over live alone, and their isolation can depress their appetite. Moreover, disabilities from osteoporosis and other diseases make it more difficult for individuals to prepare healthy meals even if they can afford to do so.

Older people are also more likely to be housebound or in convalescent homes, or to be bedridden, which dramatically fuels bone loss. In one way or another, these conditions result in reduced exposure to sunlight and a reduction in weight-bearing activities, both of which worsen bone health. In addition, medications commonly used by older citizens, such as laxatives or diuretics, inhibit calcium absorption, again worsening bone health.

These complications seem overwhelming, but there are some straightforward solutions. Ask your pharmacist about the effects of your medications on the calcium you ingest or excrete, and find out about alternative therapies that may not have the same negative effects. Request physical therapy, whether in your own home, a home with others, or a medical center. A physical therapist can choose safe but helpful exercises for you to do. Get outdoors as much as possible. If you are in a wheelchair or otherwise need assistance, ask for help getting outdoors. And, finally, take a good look at your diet to see if it is in line with the recommendations contained in this book. Share what you learn from this book with local Meals-on-Wheels programs serving the elderly in your community.

Chapter Four

Sources of Calcium

We all need calcium every day throughout our life. Calcium is necessary not only for strong bones but for many other vital functions in the body. It helps blood clot, the heart beat, and muscles move. Our teeth would decay without calcium, and our cells and nerves could not work properly. Calcium-rich diets have also played an important role in lowering blood pressure, and some evidence indicates the mineral can help prevent colon cancer. Our bodies use and contain more calcium than any other mineral.

Virtually all of the calcium in the body is stored in the skeleton. Yet this mineral is so important to the rest of the body that the body will sacrifice bone to ensure that it has enough for the other functions. Remember that the skeleton "banks" ingested calcium in order to achieve peak bone mass; the richer your calcium bank account, the more comfortable will be your retirement, when your body begins to make withdrawals from your bones. Another way to put it is that consuming enough calcium will help keep you in **positive calcium balance.**

That means you take in and absorb more calcium than you lose. Negative calcium balance occurs when you lose more calcium than you take in.

Calcium-Consumption Recommendations

If you are to stay in positive calcium balance, nutritionists at the Stedman Center recommend that you consume 1,000 to 1,500 milligrams of calcium daily, depending on your stage of life, risk for osteoporosis, and lifestyle. A serving of calcium is 300 milligrams, the amount in one cup (eight ounces) of skim milk. Thus, you should eat three to five servings of calcium-rich foods every day. Three servings provide approximately 900 milligrams of calcium—in a well-balanced diet, another 100 milligrams or so will come from the other foods you eat.

Stedman Center recommendations are in accord with the 1994 guidelines established by the National Institutes of Health Consensus Panel on Optimal Calcium Intake, the most up-to-date and reliable official statement regarding calcium consumption. The National Osteoporosis Foundation (NOF) also calls for 1,000 milligrams of calcium a day for premenopausal women and 1,500 milligrams daily for postmenopausal women not taking estrogen. The Reference Daily Intakes (RDI) created by the FDA for use in conjunction with its new nutritional-labeling system (see chapter eight) also currently call for 1,000 milligrams of calcium daily.

Our recommendations exceed the government RDA (Recommended Daily Allowance) of 800 milligrams daily. The RDA was based on studies in younger people. Stedman Center nutritionists and others have recognized that the 800-milligram allowance is insufficient for the needs of most individuals, especially older people.

Stedman Center Guidelines
for Daily Calcium Intake*

	Amount mg/day
Children and Young Adults	
1–10 years	800–1,200
11–24 years	1,200–1,500
Adult Women	
Pregnant & lactating	1,200–1,500
25–49 years (premenopausal)	1,000
50–64 years (postmenopausal)	
taking estrogen	1,000
not taking estrogen	1,500
65+ years	1,500
Adult Men	
25–64 years	1,000
65+ years	1,500

*These recommendations are based on the conclusions of the 1994 National Institutes of Health Consensus Panel on Optimal Calcium Intake.

The amount of dietary calcium necessary to prevent bone loss varies according to age, lifestyle, and many other factors. For example, as shown in the accompanying chart, during pregnancy and breast-feeding, when the baby's growth is fed by the mother, women need 50 percent more calcium than nonpregnant women of the same age. In much the same way, women who have reduced estrogen levels because of menopause or surgery in which the ovaries were removed require more calcium. Unlike pregnant and breast-feeding women, they often do not have estrogen or youth to promote the rebuilding of their bones. The matter rests even more critically on calcium.

Putting Dairy in Your Diet

The easiest way to meet your daily calcium needs through diet alone is by eating dairy products, including low-fat milk, yogurt, cheese, and ice cream or frozen yogurt. Dairy products are the most concentrated sources of calcium available as whole foods. A cup of skim milk contains 300 milligrams of calcium (the equivalent of one serving) and is usually fortified with 400 IU of vitamin D, which is the RDA for this vitamin. A single serving of fruit yogurt (one cup) contains 345 milligrams of calcium, making it tough to beat as a calcium source.

What's in a Serving?

Count one eight-ounce cup of milk as a serving.

Common portions of some dairy products and their milk equivalents in calcium are:

1 cup plain yogurt	= 1 cup milk
1 ounce Cheddar or Swiss cheese	= ¾ cup milk
1-inch cube Cheddar or Swiss cheese	= ½ cup milk
1 ounce processed cheese food	= ½ cup milk
½ cup ice cream	= ⅓ cup milk
1 tablespoon or ½ ounce processed cheese spread	= ¼ cup milk
1 tablespoon Parmesan cheese	= ¼ cup milk
½ cup cottage cheese	= ¼ cup milk

Milk

Choose skim milk, which contains no grams of fat. Whole milk by law must be 3.3 percent fat and so contains eight grams of fat per cup. Each gram of fat has nine calories, so 72 of the 150 calories (50 percent) in one cup of whole milk come from fat. By selecting a low-fat milk, which is 1 or 2 percent fat, or, better yet, skim milk, which contains less than 1 percent fat, you can avoid the excess fat, including saturated fat, in whole milk.

Children should be given whole milk until they are about two years old. At that point, you can consider switching them to 1 to 2 percent milk. Serve them milk as low in fat as they will accept; it is far better for children to drink whole milk than none at all.

Calcium Comparison Among Kinds of Milk Serving Size = One Cup			
	Calories	Calcium (mg)	Fat (g)
Skim	86	302	0
Low-fat:			
1 percent	102	300	2
2 percent	121	297	4
Whole (3.3 percent fat)	150	291	8
Buttermilk (4 percent fat)	99	285	2

Cheese

Most cheese is packed with calcium, like the milk that it comes from. But it can be equally packed with unhealthy stuff, particularly saturated fat and sodium. Too much fat can lead to high cholesterol levels and weight problems. Too much sodium contributes to the development of hypertension, which leads to stroke and, most important for those concerned with osteoporosis, increases the urinary excretion of calcium. The advent of low-fat/non-fat/low-sodium processing of cheeses and other dairy products has changed our thinking about nutrition choices and reduces many people's need for calcium supplementation.

There is a wide variety of such cheeses on the market today. If they are used in recipes, any difference in taste or consistency will never be noticed in the finished product. For instance, replacing whole-milk ricotta with low-fat or nonfat ricotta in lasagna is an excellent-tasting substitution and makes a healthful, high-calcium, low-fat meal.

If you find yourself disappointed with the taste of these alternative cheeses, you can try mixing a little bit of a tastier, high-fat cheese with low-fat cheeses in a recipe to retain the flavor you like while cutting down on fat. Just as it may take a while to wean yourself off whole milk, it may take a while to acquire a taste for low-fat or nonfat cheese. Once you acquire a taste for it and feel better, you won't want to go back.

Of course, not all cheese is created equal when it comes to calcium content. A ½-cup serving of ricotta, for instance, weighs in at 340 milligrams of calcium, whereas an equal amount of creamed cottage cheese provides a relatively paltry 50 milligrams. It is helpful to know the calcium content of the different cheeses because they can be combined in a variety of ways with other foods to create a variety of calcium-rich meals. When shopping, use the chart on pages 41–42 to determine the calcium and fat content of various cheeses.

Yogurt

Yogurt is another calcium-rich food that has become increasingly popular in recent years. It comes in numerous flavors, styles, and brands. Some yogurts are creamy, and some contain chunks of fruit on the bottom. Flavors range from strawberry mango to cappuccino. The readily available single-serving containers make yogurt a convenient item for a calcium-rich bagged lunch or snack.

Yogurt, like cheese, can contain a significant amount of fat, but most varieties available today are low-fat and contain only two to three grams of fat per serving. Some are nonfat. Sugar-free yogurt containing aspartame is another low calorie option.

The various brands and styles of yogurt contain different amounts of calcium. The best sources of calcium among the wide range of yogurt styles now on the market are Dannon Light or Dannon Fruit on the Bottom, weighing in at 350 milligrams of calcium apiece. The former is a healthier choice, because it contains 150 calories and no fat, versus 240 calories and three grams of fat for the latter. At the low end of the calcium scale sits low fat Jell-O Jigglers Bits & Yogurt; a six-ounce serving features 150 milligrams of calcium, 1.5 grams of fat, and 220 calories or more.

Frozen yogurt, a tasty, less fattening alternative to ice cream, typically contains about twice as much calcium and considerably less fat (see the chart on page 40).

Calcium and Fat Comparison Among Yogurt, Frozen Yogurt, and Ice Cream (Serving Size = One Cup)

	Calcium (mg)	Fat (g)	Calories
Yogurt			
regular	300–400	5	240–270
low-fat	300–400	2–3	150–270
nonfat	250–300	0	100
Frozen Yogurt			
low-fat	300–400	2.3	200–250
nonfat	300	0	100
Ice Cream			
regular	194	14.1	257
low-fat	204	6.7	199
soft-serve	273	8.4	266
Sherbet	104	3.8	270

Nondairy Sources of Calcium

In addition to dairy foods, we get a fair amount of calcium from other food groups: fruits and vegetables, 9 percent; meat, 9 percent; grain, 4 percent; and other foods, 2 percent. All together, that accounts for almost a quarter of the daily calcium intake in a typical diet.

One cup of broccoli, for instance, contains 177 milligrams of calcium, about half the amount in the same quantity of yogurt. Four ounces of tofu contain 108 milligrams, and three ounces of canned shrimp contain 98 milligrams, equivalent to about a third of a cup of milk. Most meats contain only trace amounts of calcium, but 13 to 19 oysters offer 226 milligrams! Combination foods

Calcium Content of Cheese

Food	Serving Size	Calcium	Calories	Fat	Saturated Fat
		(mg)		(g)	(g)
Alpine Lace Mozzarella	¼ cup grated	188	71	4	3
American cheese	1 slice	107	80	7	4
Blue cheese	1-inch cube	91	61	5	3
Borden Lite-Line	1 slice	188	40	2	1
Brie cheese	1-inch cube	66	51	4	3
Camembert cheese	1-inch cube	66	51	4	3
Cheddar cheese	1-inch cube	90	69	6	4
Cheese Whiz, mild	¼ cup	359	195	14	9
Cheshire cheese	1-inch cube	126	64	5	3
Colby cheese	1-inch cube	90	69	6	4
Cottage cheese, regular	½ cup	63	109	5	3
Cottage cheese, low-fat (2-percent milk)	½ cup	77	101	2	1
Cream cheese, regular	1 tablespoon	12	51	5	3
Cream cheese, light	1 tablespoon	20	32	3	2
Farmer cheese, solid	1-inch cube	126	64	5	3
Feta cheese	1-inch cube	84	45	4	3
Fontina cheese	1-inch cube	108	55	5	3
Goat cheese	1-inch cube	84	45	4	3

Calcium Content of Cheese *(cont'd.)*

Food	Serving Size	Calcium	Calories	Fat	Saturated Fat
		(mg)		(g)	(g)
Gouda cheese	1-inch cube	124	61	5	3
Gruyère cheese	1-inch cube	144	56	4	3
Havarti cheese	1-inch cube	91	70	6	4
Hickory Farms Port Wine cold pack	1-inch cube	87	58	4	3
Kraft Free Singles	1 slice	123	25	0	0
Liederkranz	1-inch cube	91	61	5	3
Monterey Jack cheese	1-inch cube	123	63	5	3
Mozzarella cheese, part-skim	½ cup grated	413	158	10	6
Muenster cheese	1-inch cube	126	64	5	3
Parmesan cheese, dry	1 tablespoon	69	23	2	1
Parmesan cheese, fresh hard	1-inch cube	142	47	3	2
Port du Salut cheese	1-inch cube	123	63	5	3
Pot cheese	¼ cup	20	53	0	0
Provolone cheese	1-inch cube	124	61	3	5
Ricotta cheese, whole-milk	½ cup	255	214	16	10
Ricotta cheese, part-skim	½ cup	335	170	10	6
Romano cheese	1 tablespoon	69	23	2	1
Roquefort cheese	1-inch cube	91	61	5	3
String cheese	1 stick	168	64	4	3
Swiss cheese	1-inch cube	144	56	4	3

made with ingredients from more than one food group —such as pizza or macaroni and cheese—make excellent sources of calcium in the context of other foods, but watch out for the fat. Collards, kale, mustard greens, and turnip greens are vegetables with relatively high calcium contents—choose them from the cafeteria line or the market.

Besides the wide variety of dairy products and other foods that naturally contain high amounts of calcium, increasing numbers of food manufacturers are adding calcium to foods such as fruit juice, flour, cereal, and breakfast bars. Such products can boost your daily calcium intake while helping you balance your diet. Look at labels and ingredient lists for supplement claims and information.

Calcium Supplements

Ideally, you can meet all your calcium needs from foods in a carefully selected diet. People who find it difficult to take in several glasses of milk or the equivalent in calcium every day, however, will find calcium supplements in the form of pills, chewable tablets, or liquids a valuable way to increase calcium intake.

You may already be getting a small amount of calcium, usually about 100 milligrams, as well as vitamin D in a multivitamin. If you find that you need more supplemental calcium than that, you should buy a special supplement, available in any pharmacy. You must consider the type of supplement, the amount of calcium it contains, how digestible it is, and how much it costs.

Some supplements contain more calcium than others. Supplements are sold under many brand names, but you also should read their ingredients label to determine the actual percentage of calcium they contain, which is usually called **elemental calcium.** The label will tell you what kind of calcium the supplement contains. As you can see by the accompanying table, the amount of elemental calcium in supplements varies by as much as 31 percent.

Comparison of Percentage of Elemental Calcium in Supplements	
Type	% Calcium
Calcium carbonate	40
Calcium chloride	36
Calcium phosphate	30
Oyster shell	28
Calcium citrate	21
Calcium lactate	13
Calcium gluconate	9

The most commonly used supplement is calcium carbonate, which is available as chewing gum or chewable tablets. The best-known brand name for calcium carbonate is Tums, often used as an antacid pill. Each chewable tablet contains from 200 to 500 milligrams of elemental calcium.

Some types of calcium are better absorbed by the body than others. You can be sure that the supplement you buy absorbs well if one of the tablets dissolves almost entirely in a small glass of warm water or vinegar within 30 minutes. *Your calcium supplement should contain no aluminum because aluminum reduces calcium absorption.*

Overall, supplemental calcium is best absorbed when taken in small amounts. If you want to take a supplement that contains 500 milligrams a day, taking one tablet is appropriate. If you're taking more than that, it is better to split it up into doses of 250 milligrams apiece.

Establish a daily time or times to take your supplement and plan to take it with or immediately following a meal, which tends to increase absorption. Do not take it with food that is very high in fiber, such as a high-fiber breakfast cereal, or with any bulk-forming laxative such as Metamucil: fiber can reduce your calcium absorption. Drinking plenty of fluids while taking calcium supplements will help increase absorption. You can also enhance the absorption of your calcium supplement by taking it with foods high in vitamin C, like fruits and vegetables.

Do not take an iron supplement at the same time as calcium, because the calcium will inhibit its absorption. If you need to take both supplements, take them at different times—for instance, iron after breakfast and calcium after dinner.

Do not take supplements that contain bone meal or dolomite; although they are high in calcium (one teaspoon of dolomite contains 1,180 milligrams of calcium), they may contain unsafe amounts of lead, cadmium, and/or other toxic metals. Again, we recommend smaller doses throughout the day and in conjunction with a calcium-rich diet.

Calcium supplements may cause side effects. The most common are gas, intestinal irritation, constipation, or nausea in people with too little stomach acid. These people may be better off with the more expensive calcium-citrate pills, which are gentler on the stomach.

Always check with your pharmacist to make sure that your supplements will not cause side effects by interacting with any prescription drugs you take.

Of course, as a consumer of supplements, one should

be wary of false advertising or questionable health claims. For instance, no one nutrient or drug can cure osteoporosis, so do not be taken in by any such claims. Since calcium and vitamin-D supplements (like all vitamin and mineral supplements) are considered neither a food nor a drug, they are unregulated by the FDA or the Department of Agriculture. That means you cannot be guaranteed that their health claims are valid. Be cautious when choosing them.

One potential complication of supplements is that calcium consumption above 2,000 milligrams daily puts you at risk for kidney stones and increased blood calcium, which can lead to serious problems. Since to approach that level of calcium consumption you would have to drink a gallon of milk or the equivalent a day, excessive calcium is a potential problem virtually only among people taking supplements. Remember, you do not need to take a 1,000-milligram calcium supplement if you are already drinking three glasses of milk daily; that would raise your calcium intake to about 1,900 milligrams a day, more than anyone needs. *As the name says, use these tablets only to supplement your dietary calcium.*

Are You Getting Enough Calcium?

Answer these questions according to what you ate yesterday to count your calcium. Enter your scores in the box at the end of each question.

1. Did you drink milk (regular, low-fat, or skim) yesterday? If so, give yourself four points for every eight-ounce glass (one cup).   _____
2. Did you eat fruit yogurt? Give yourself four points for every cup.   _____

3. Did you drink juice fortified with calcium? Give yourself four points for every eight-ounce glass. _____

4. Did you eat cereal with one-half cup of milk? For every serving, give yourself two points. _____

5. Did you have some cheese (American, Swiss, Cheddar)? For every two slices (one ounce), give yourself two points. _____

6. Did you eat canned salmon with bones? If you had three ounces (a regular-sized can), give yourself two points _____

7. Did you eat a one-half-cup serving of frozen yogurt? Give yourself two points _____

8. Did you eat broccoli, kale, collards, or bok choy? If you had one-half cup of one of these vegetables, give yourself one point. _____

9. Did you have some cottage cheese? If you ate one-half cup of the low-fat or creamed variety, give yourself one point. _____

10. Did you eat some ice cream? If you ate one-half cup, give yourself one point. _____

Add up your points and enter the total score here: _____

If you need four servings of calcium and scored 16 points, congratulations—you are getting enough calcium in your diet. If you are not getting enough calcium, read chapter five to find out how adding more dairy food or other calcium-rich foods can make a big difference in your diet.

Maximizing Calcium Utilization

In addition to consuming enough calcium, you can help your body maximize its ability to absorb calcium. This will help ensure that you stay in positive calcium balance. Normally, the body absorbs only 10 to 30 percent of the calcium you ingest. (RDI's are based on maximum normal absorption, and not on 100 percent absorption.) Many factors influence how successfully your body maintains its calcium bank account.

The most important factor is vitamin D.

Vitamin D and Calcium Absorption

Vitamin D plays a fundamental role in calcium absorption and bone health. The body cannot absorb calcium or make new bone without it. Vitamin D facilitates calcium absorption in the intestine by a complex mechanism that scientists have only recently begun to understand.

Imagine vitamin D as a key that unlocks a door to your body, allowing calcium to leave the intestine and enter the bloodstream. Vitamin D also helps reclaim calcium in the kidneys, where calcium is filtered and prepared for excretion in the urine.

The body gets vitamin D in two ways. It is naturally synthesized in the skin upon exposure to ultraviolet radiation from sunlight. That's why it's called the "sunshine vitamin." How much vitamin D you produce depends upon how long you are out in the sun; in general, at least 15 minutes of exposure per day is required to create the 400 IU required for normal body function. Many factors, however, can modulate the effects of sun exposure, including the time of year and time of day when you are outside and the clothes you wear. Many people now put on sunscreen before going outside, to avoid harmful overexposure to ultraviolet rays. But sunscreen also blocks vitamin-D absorption. So if you wear sunscreen all of the time you are outdoors or do not have regular exposure to the sun, you must depend upon the other source for vitamin D to meet your body's need: diet.

Though most people are able to obtain enough vitamin D naturally, many studies show that vitamin-D production decreases in the elderly, in people who are housebound, and during winter. Elderly people in convalescent homes, who are unable to get outside, are at high risk for vitamin-D deficiency. Some people may require vitamin-D supplements to achieve the RDA of 400 IU. Most multivitamins do contain 400 IU of vitamin D.

Vitamin D is found in eggs, butter, liver, and fatty fish (such as mackerel). Milk is usually fortified with vitamin D, so all dairy products are a rich source of this vitamin. One cup of fortified milk provides about 100 IU of vitamin D. Check the nutrition label on the milk you buy to make sure it is supplemented with vitamin D.

Vitamin D, whether you get it from the sun, from the food you eat, and/or from supplements, circulates in the blood, where it is activated to a form that is responsible for modulating calcium absorption from the intestine, as well as other functions. Vitamin-D activation has two steps. First the liver changes vitamin D into an intermediary factor, called calcidiol. Then from calcidiol the kidneys produce the active vitamin-D metabolite, calcitriol.

Parathyroid-Gland Activity

The parathyroid glands also play an important role in how well your body absorbs calcium. Located in the neck, around the windpipe, these glands regulate the calcium level in the body through a complicated system that makes sure adequate calcium is available for the multiple body functions that depend on the mineral.

When calcium levels in the blood dip below adequate levels, the parathyroid glands initiate the bone-remodeling process described in chapter one. The four tiny glands at the base of the thyroid release a hormone that stimulates the bone-destroying osteoclast cells. These cells carve holes in bone, and the calcium contained in those bones escapes into the blood. The less circulating calcium available, the more bone is broken down. If you do not eat or absorb enough calcium, the parathyroid glands direct mobilization of calcium from your bones to ensure normal body functions.

Bone remodeling is a natural process, and in people with adequate calcium levels before they achieve peak bone mass, the body is able to build more than enough new bone to replace bone destroyed in this way. But as described earlier, older people, particularly post-menopausal women, tend to lose more bone than is replaced. The less calcium provided by the diet, the swifter the bone loss. It is estimated that 25 years in negative calcium balance consumes one-third of the human skeleton.

Reduced estrogen levels leave women even more vulnerable to the bone-dissolving actions of parathyroid hormones. Estrogen helps block parathyroid stimulation. When estrogen levels fall after menopause, the low levels of parathyroid hormone that previously would not have led to bone loss begin to stimulate bone breakdown. One of the purposes of estrogen-replacement therapy is to slow the parathyroid stimulus.

Complicating matters further, parathyroid hormone activity increases as we get older. This increase further stimulates bone-destroying osteoclast cells.

Calcitonin

The hormone calcitonin is released by the thyroid gland, which surrounds the parathyroid. Calcitonin plays a role in bone maintenance. It inhibits the bone-destroying activity of the osteoclasts. Calcitonin levels decrease with age, another reason we lose bone as we get older. Although estrogen stimulates calcitonin secretion, researchers are unsure whether menopause actually lowers calcitonin levels. They do know that women with osteoporosis have less calcitonin than women who do not, and that all women have less calcitonin than men, who have greater bone mass. As discussed in chapter two, calcitonin is available as a prescription drug by injection to people with osteoporosis.

Phosphorus

Phosphorus is another mineral crucial for bone health. Your body cannot make bone without it. The ratio of phosphorus to calcium in the body also affects bone metabolism. The ideal ratio between phosphorus and calcium is 1:1. Phosphorus is found in almost all foods and does not need supplementation or enhancement in the diet. On the contrary, maintaining a 1:1 ratio is diffi-cult not only because we ingest too little calcium but also because we typically ingest too much phosphorus.

Calcium Inhibitors

Maintaining a positive calcium balance depends partly on how well your body absorbs calcium. We already talked about the key role of vitamin D in facilitating cal-cium absorption. But some substances are enemies of calcium. Many of these are also enemies of good nutri-tion.

Salt, caffeine, and alcohol, among other substances, can increase the excretion rate of calcium through the urine, robbing you of the calcium you consume.

Salt

Americans consume excessive amounts of salt (sodium), much of it hidden in fast foods, convenience foods, and processed foods. The Stedman Center recommends you eat no more than 3,300 milligrams of salt daily. If you ingest too much salt, calcium that your body needs will be released into your urine.

Low-sodium diets are associated with decreased bone loss. Scientists believe a low-salt diet may slow osteo-porosis by helping the body retain calcium that normally would be excreted in the urine.

Another reason to watch your sodium intake is that, though sodium is an essential element, too much can also increase your risk for hypertension. Instead of salt, use spices such as garlic or basil if you want to add extra flavor to your food. You may also wean yourself off ex-cessive salt by gradually using salt substitutes that con-tain no sodium.

Caffeine

Drinking excessive amounts of caffeinated coffee or tea in a day can also cause significant urinary calcium loss. Several studies show that up to 31 percent of postmenopausal women with significant bone loss drink four or more cups of coffee per day; in contrast, only 19 percent of women with normal bone drank that much coffee. Colas and some other soft drinks also contain high amounts of caffeine. The Stedman Center recommends limiting all caffeinated beverages to two to three cups a day. Consider switching to decaffeinated coffee or tea, hot chocolate, lemonade, fruit juice, skim milk, or plain old water instead of caffeinated beverages.

Alcohol

Alcohol provides empty calories and effectively suppresses the appetite, which decreases intake of essential vitamins, minerals, and nutritional foods. Alcoholics, who typically are malnourished, are at high risk for osteoporosis. Alcohol impairs intestinal calcium absorption when used in excess and should not be ingested along with your calcium sources. If you drink alcohol, you should limit your intake to one or two servings a day, less if you are at risk for osteoporosis. One serving equals a 12-ounce beer, a four-ounce glass of wine, or 1.5 to two ounces of liquor.

Nicotine

You can add bone loss to the long list of dangerous effects that smoking cigarettes has on the body. Indeed, many studies have associated smoking with bone loss and osteoporosis. In general, the more cigarettes a person smokes over his or her lifetime, the lower the bone mass.

Stress

Another calcium robber is an invisible assailant: stress. Stress can make the body more susceptible to illness and may impair the immune system. It also decreases calcium absorption and increases calcium loss through urine excretion. When you are under stress, it is especially important that you get enough calcium.

Excessive Protein

The body needs protein to function, but Americans eat far more protein than is good for them, especially meat and whole-milk cheese, which are high in saturated fat. Saturated fat is associated with high cholesterol, which contributes to a number of chronic diseases. Americans eat 10 times as much meat as do the Chinese, and the death rate due to heart disease among American men is about 17 times higher than that of Chinese men of the same age. Research shows there is a correlation between the high meat consumption of Americans, with the associated high levels of saturated fat, and the high rate of heart disease.

Another important reason not to eat too much meat is that it appears to be harmful to healthy bones. Swift bone loss results from excessive protein intake. One study showed that women whose average daily protein intake was 65 grams, or about three hamburgers per day, excreted an extra 26 milligrams of calcium per day in their urine. Over one year, such calcium loss will probably result in a decrease in bone mass of 1 percent.

You do not have to abstain from eating meat altogether, but you should eat it in moderation. The Stedman Center recommends total daily consumption of three to six ounces of meat, which equals one to two servings, each of them about the size of a deck of cards. That means eating about half as much meat as Americans typically consume.

Protein is an essential part of the diet, however, and a deficit can cause debilitating disease. Fortunately, you can also get protein from other sources. Excellent low-fat alternatives to regular meat products include lean beef, poultry (especially turkey or chicken white meat without skin), lean fish, dry beans, egg whites, and dairy products. The National Academy of Sciences recommends that women eat 50 grams of protein daily, men 63 grams. The U.S. Department of Agriculture says that adults can ingest sufficient protein by eating two to three servings a day of 2.5 to three ounces each of protein-rich foods.

Oxalates

Foods that contain oxalates combine with dietary calcium in the intestines and prevent its absorption. Oxalates can be found in:

• asparagus	• peanuts
• beets	• rhubarb
• chives	• sorrel
• cocoa	• spinach
• dandelion greens	• summer squash
• green beans	• Swiss chard
• parsley	• tea

Oxalic acid holds calcium in the intestine and makes it unavailable to the rest of the body. Even though a cup of cooked spinach contains 242 milligrams of calcium, your body will be unable to use the calcium efficiently, so do not depend on it as a good calcium source. Vegetables that contain calcium and are low in oxalic acid include endives, kale, and turnip greens.

Foods containing oxalates may exacerbate a lack of calcium in people who have trouble absorbing enough calcium, such as the elderly. Although you do not need to eliminate foods containing oxalates from your diet, if you are having trouble maintaining adequate calcium levels you should avoid foods containing oxalates during meals in which you are consuming calcium products. To maximize your calcium consumption, wait several hours between the consumption of calcium-rich foods and any products containing oxalates to avoid their neutralizing effect on calcium absorption.

Phytates

Phytates are phosphorus compounds found in bran or oatmeal and in legumes, which include dried beans and peas. Like oxalates, they also bind with dietary calcium in the intestines. You cannot count on the milk in a bowl of oatmeal or bran cereal as part of your calcium intake, for the phytates those cereals contain will prevent its absorption. You can eat cereals that contain bran or oatmeal for fiber, but separate this from your high-calcium meals. And, as with oxalates, eat dried beans or dried peas separately from meals that you depend upon for calcium.

Excessive Fiber

Much has been written about the importance of sufficient dietary fiber—carbohydrates found in plant foods such as bran, brown rice, fruits and vegetables, and whole-wheat bread. Fiber aids digestion, lowers cholesterol levels, and reduces the risk of colon cancer. Yet too much fiber can speed digestion to the point where minerals such as calcium are not properly absorbed by the body. Excessively high fiber intake—more than 30 grams a day—contributes to bone loss and is not recommended for anyone at risk for osteoporosis.

Vitamin D

Too little vitamin D doesn't inhibit calcium absorption, but it can cause other serious problems in your bones.

Also, you may have a vitamin-D deficiency if something interferes with your activation process, or if you suffer from liver or kidney disease. The deficiency will occur no matter how much sunlight you are exposed to or how much vitamin D you eat or take in pill form.

Severe vitamin-D deficiency can cause **osteomalacia** in adults and children and also **rickets** in children. These disorders are the result of soft bones that occur when the body fails to provide enough calcium (or phosphorus) to harden bones because of vitamin-D deficiency. Osteomalacia in adults is different from the bone losing disease, osteoporosis. Although it resembles osteoporosis in X-rays and can cause fractures in some people, osteomalacia in most forms may be cured by administration of vitamin D or an active metabolite of vitamin D. In contrast, vitamin D and its metabolites cannot cure osteoporosis but may only slow the bone loss the disease causes.

Vitamin D can, however, be too much of a good thing, and excessive amounts of it can actually increase bone loss. Intake of vitamin D beyond 800 IU should only be done under the supervision of a doctor.

Chapter Six

Calcium for the Lactose-Intolerant

Lactose intolerance means a person has difficulty digesting the sugar in dairy products, which is called **lactose.** This carbohydrate is made up of two sugars—glucose and galactose. The most common reason people are lactose-intolerant is that they lack sufficient **lactase,** an intestinal enzyme that breaks down lactose into the two digestible sugars.

People with low lactase may experience diarrhea, stomach cramps, gas, and bloating after eating products containing lactose, because the sugar passes through their digestive system without being absorbed or digested. Symptoms usually occur 15 to 30 minutes after consuming a dairy food.

An estimated 30 million Americans are lactose-intolerant, including nearly a quarter of all Caucasian Americans and more than three-quarters of African Americans, who for poorly understood reasons are at high risk of developing the condition. Asians, Eskimos, Jews, Native Americans, and Hispanics also are at high risk. The condition is more frequent in the elderly because the body gradually makes less lactase as we age, although heredity may cause some children to lose their ability to produce lactase by the time they start elementary school. Sometimes infants are born with **alactasia,** or congenital lactose intolerance, or with a birth defect known as **galactosemia,** in which the baby lacks the enzyme to convert galactose into glucose. Both conditions are serious and require immediate attention; however, both are treatable if detected early.

Symptoms

You may be lactose-intolerant if you feel bloated or experience other symptoms for up to 12 hours after drinking a cup of milk. Try avoiding dairy foods for a few days to see if the symptoms go away. If they do not, see your doctor; those symptoms may indicate the presence of a different disease. If the symptoms go away, drink a glass of milk. Should the symptoms recur, you may well be lactose-intolerant. Your doctor can confirm whether you are, through laboratory tests.

The **lactose-tolerance test** involves drinking a large glass of a sweet drink laced with 50 grams of lactose. Blood is drawn periodically to see if the blood-glucose level rises. If it fails to rise, the body is not digesting the lactose and absorbing the resulting glucose.

The **hydrogen-breath test** analyzes exhaled breath to see if it contains hydrogen after you drink a sweet, lactose-loaded drink. The presence of hydrogen indicates the presence of undigested lactose, which ferments into several gases, including hydrogen.

Managing Lactose Intolerance

People with lactose intolerance can maintain calcium intake in several ways. They can eat more tolerable dairy foods with relatively low lactose content, choose calcium-fortified foods or other sources of dietary calcium, take calcium supplements, or change their eating habits so that, for instance, they drink milk with a meal or with other foods, which alleviates the symptoms. The vast majority of people who are lactose-intolerant do not have to abandon dairy foods. They do have to change their milk-drinking habits in varying degrees, depending upon the severity of their symptoms. A doctor can help you determine your level of lactose intolerance. Safe, inexpensive pills and liquids on the market can also make milk digestible. Yet some people, unaware of how they can continue to enjoy milk, mistakenly curtail their milk drinking severely.

The danger for people who are lactose-intolerant is that they will not consume enough calcium, since dairy products generally supply more than three-quarters of calcium, the most important mineral in your body. Milk is also an important source of protein, vitamin A, B vitamins, and riboflavin.

Milk products are not only the most abundant calcium source, but also the most delicious. Tolerance levels vary widely, yet few lactose-intolerant people know how much milk they can tolerate.

Four out of five people with low lactase levels can drink a cup of milk with a meal without having symptoms. Although some people with low lactase levels experience symptoms after drinking very little milk, others can drink several glasses with no pain or gas.

Low-Lactose Cheeses

Most people can also eat some kinds of cheese without difficulty. People with lactose intolerance, however, must be careful when they choose cheese for a meal. The whey family of cheeses, for instance, contains large amounts of lactose. This family includes cottage cheese and ricotta cheese, which contain seven or eight grams of lactose per cup. But other cheeses, primarily the hard, aged cheeses, contain less than one gram of lactose per ounce because much of the milk sugar is removed during processing.

Alternative Dairy Products

Soy milk offers another nutritious way to get calcium in your diet without ingesting lactose. Make sure you select a brand that is fortified with calcium. Unfortified soy milk (made from soybeans) naturally contains only about 55 milligrams of calcium per cup. Calcium-fortified brands, however, make the calcium level equal to that in a cup of dairy milk.

Low-lactose milk and acidophilus milk are other alternatives for obtaining dietary calcium that are now available in most dairy coolers. These kinds of milk contain about 70 percent less lactose than regular milk but just as much calcium. Orange juice fortified with calcium also provides as much of the mineral as a cup of skim milk. Bread fortified with calcium is another rich source of calcium for the lactose-intolerant.

Eat yogurt with acidophilus-bacteria cultures, since it contains lactase, which will break down the lactose. Be aware that yogurts are fortified with nonfat milk solids and they can contain as much lactose as milk. Read the list of ingredients to see if a particular brand of yogurt contains nonfat milk solids.

If your lactose intolerance is so severe you cannot tolerate enough milk to meet your daily calcium requirement, you may also take calcium supplements. Avoid supplements made of calcium lactate, which, as the name implies, contain lactose. Products made from calcium carbonate and calcium phosphate are lactose-free.

Lactase-Enzyme Products

Another way to deal with lactose intolerance is to use any of the lactase-enzyme preparations that are available at your local pharmacy. The enzyme is a protein that can be added to milk, where it divides the lactose into the digestible sugars glucose and galactose. Normally that breakdown occurs in the intestines. The lactase-treated milk does the job for the body, so the two sugars can then be easily absorbed by the body.

If you add the liquid lactase enzyme to a quart of milk ahead of time, it will be ready to drink in about 24 hours. You can adjust the amount according to your tolerance level. Once milk is treated with a commercial enzyme, you can use it as you would normally use milk in any recipe that calls for milk.

The lactase-treated milk holds the same nutritional value as does regular milk, although the lactase-treated milk tastes sweeter than regular milk, because glucose and galactose are sweeter than lactose. But the only real difference between the two kinds of milk is that the lactase-treated milk is more digestible.

At most supermarkets you can also buy milk in which the lactase enzyme has already been added. Other than the lactase enzyme, nothing is added or subtracted from the lactase-treated milk, so it has the same nutritional value as untreated milk. The list of other lactase-treated dairy products and low-lactose milks now sold at supermarkets is growing, including cottage cheese.

The lactase enzyme is also available as a tablet you can take just before you eat foods that contain lactose, such as cheese lasagna. The lactase enzyme in the tablet breaks down the lactose in the stomach into the two digestible sugars. Two of the more commonly known brand names are Lactaid and Dairy Ease. Though enzyme tablets make eating more expensive, they allow many lactose-intolerant people to eat as many dairy foods as they want when they want. These tablets are sold in pharmacies and supermarkets.

Lactose Content of Dairy Foods		
Product	Unit	Grams of Lactose
Milks		
Buttermilk	1 cup	9–11
Chocolate milk	1 cup	10–12
Dried whole milk	1 cup	48
Eggnog	1 cup	14
Evaporated milk	1 cup	20
Goat's milk	1 cup	9.4
Human milk	1 cup	13.8
Low-fat milk	1 cup	9–13
Low-sodium milk	1 cup	9
Nonfat dry milk	1 cup	40
Skim milk	1 cup	12–14
Sweetened condensed milk	1 cup	35
Whole milk	1 cup	11
Miscellaneous Dairy Foods		
Butter	1 teaspoon	.06
Butter	2 pats	.10
Half and Half	1 tablespoon	0.6
Light cream	1 tablespoon	0.6
Low-fat yogurt	1 cup	10–15
Margarine	1 teaspoon	.90
Sour cream	½ cup	3.2
Cheeses		
American processed cheese	1 ounce	.50
Blue cheese	1 ounce	.70

Lactose Content of Dairy Foods *(cont'd.)*		
Product	Unit	Grams of Lactose
Cheeses (cont'd.)		
Camembert	1 ounce	.10
Cheddar	1 ounce	.50
Colby	1 ounce	.70
Cottage cheese	1 cup	5–6
Cream cheese	1 ounce	.80
Dry-curd cottage cheese	1 cup	2
Gouda	1 ounce	.60
Limburger	1 ounce	.10
Low-fat cottage cheese	1 cup	7
Parmesan	1 ounce	.80
Pimento processed	1 ounce	.50–1.70
Swiss	1 ounce	.50

Milk Allergies

Some children cannot consume milk because they are allergic to it. Lactose intolerance is different from an allergy to milk. Milk allergies generally are considered to be a sensitivity to the protein in milk, although theories differ as to their cause. Symptoms following milk ingestion include asthma, mucus buildup, wheezing, rash, vomiting, and/or eczema. Babies who are allergic to milk are usually placed on a soy-protein formula. As they grow older, children gradually lose their allergic reaction to milk. The regimen for people with milk allergies differs from that of people who are lactose-intolerant, and experts disagree on how to treat the allergy. Children with milk allergies need alternative sources of calcium-rich foods or calcium supplements, as described in chapter four.

Chapter Seven

Capitalizing on Calcium in Cooking

Some people at risk for osteoporosis are intimidated when they learn they should consume three to five servings of calcium daily. No wonder—that equals drinking a quart of milk or more. Drinking milk is an excellent way to get calcium, but there are many other ways to add calcium to your diet using nonfat or low-fat dairy sources. They include cooking with milk, adding cheese, yogurt, or tofu to foods, choosing calcium-rich vegetables, and adding nonfat dry milk solids to recipes. Whether you are cooking for one or for an entire family, it is simple to boost the calcium in the dishes you prepare. Here are some ways to capitalize on calcium in your cooking.

Milk and Yogurt

Use skim milk fortified with nonfat milk powder to replace cream in recipes. You lose the fat but not the thickening agent.

Make hot cocoa and cream soups with skim milk

instead of water. You can get up to 300 milligrams of calcium per serving, and no fat.

Top angel-food cake, fruit, and Jell-O with nonfat flavored yogurt.

Choose calcium-rich desserts such as frozen yogurt, puddings, or custard. Serve instant pudding or custard made with skim milk to keep fat down.

Freeze milk in ice-cube trays and use it crushed in shakes you make in your blender.

Cook with nonfat plain yogurt instead of sour cream. It's a delicious substitute for calcium-poor, fat-laden sour cream atop baked potatoes and in recipes. When you eat a baked potato, substituting one-half cup of low-fat plain yogurt for butter or sour cream will add 150 milligrams of calcium but no fat to your meal.

Use yogurt as a thickener in soups, casseroles, and beverages.

Substitute nonfat plain yogurt for mayonnaise in dips and salad dressings.

Nonfat Dry Milk Solids

Nonfat dry milk solids are a simple, nutritious way to increase the calcium content in foods you cook. Each teaspoon of powdered nonfat dry milk contains 50 milligrams of calcium—and no fat. Besides boosting calcium, the substance also enhances the vitamin-D content and the taste of foods. Nonfat powdered dry milk makes casseroles creamier and soups thicker. Be creative in finding ways to add dry milk to your daily diet.

Any dish that depends upon a white sauce—such as fettuccine Alfredo—offers an opportunity to replace fatty cream with nonfat dry milk solids to boost your calcium intake without fat. Although traditional Alfredo sauce oozes fat, you can make it with skim milk, adding nonfat dry milk to thicken it.

Add a couple of tablespoons of nonfat dry milk powder to fresh skim milk, hot cereal, cold cereal, yogurt, salad dressing, creamed soups, muffins, or mashed potatoes. The ratio for mashed potatoes should be about two tablespoons to every cup of potatoes.

Add an extra one-quarter cup of nonfat milk solids to each cup of milk called for whenever you make meat loaf or cakes, muffins, or other baked goods. Two four-inch pancakes, for instance, usually contain 76 milligrams of calcium. Adding a teaspoon of nonfat dry milk to each more than doubles their calcium content.

When you cook with nonfat dry milk, combine the powder with another cold liquid and stir until the granules dissolve before adding it to the rest of the recipe, since the powder dissolves poorly in hot liquids.

Evaporated Milk

Cooking with evaporated skim milk also doubles the calcium content in food. Avoid evaporated whole milk because of its fat: it contains twice the calories and fat of regular milk. Create your own cream sauces with evaporated skim milk—try sauces flavored with Cajun seasonings or Parmesan cheese to spoon over pasta or vegetables.

Replace nondairy coffee creamers with evaporated skim milk. It is creamier than regular skim milk and tastes better than the fake stuff!

Evaporated skim milk is also a tasty, calcium-rich substitute for cream in soups and casseroles.

Cheese

Another simple way to boost your calcium consumption is to get into the habit of adding small amounts of cheese to dishes to enhance flavor and calcium content. Choose low-fat cheese or nonfat cheese whenever possible. You can mix low-fat cheese with regular cheese in recipes to retain taste yet hold down the amount of fat in your cooking. Keep in mind that most cheeses have a very strong flavor, so that just a small amount appreciably changes a dish.

Use nonfat ricotta or cottage cheese in lasagna and pasta dishes or in salads. Sprinkle salads with grated cheese. Stir shredded low-fat or nonfat cheese into creamed soups. Add shredded nonfat cheese to beaten eggs when making an omelet or scrambled eggs. Mix nonfat or low-fat cheese into mashed potatoes or rice. Melt some low-fat Cheddar- or Swiss-cheese cubes on pasta or rice. Make a simple mini-pizza by topping an English-muffin half with tomato, a spoonful of ricotta, and a sprinkling of oregano and grated Parmesan cheese, then heating until it is bubbly. Serve melted cheese, sprinkled with your favorite herb or spice, as a dip for chips and vegetables. Keep cheese soft using a fondue pot.

As a topping for cooked vegetables and other dishes, substitute a small amount of grated cheese for butter or salt. Two tablespoons of Parmesan cheese atop a dish of broccoli adds zest to the vegetables as well as 140 milligrams of calcium—and only 50 calories. In contrast, two tablespoons of butter adds 200 calories—and no calcium. Just remember to go easy on high-fat cheeses; choose low-fat varieties whenever possible, and keep your eye on the sodium levels.

Combination Foods

Dishes that incorporate foods from the milk group with foods from other groups can be excellent sources of calcium. Some of these foods may not immediately spring to mind when you are adding up calcium—such as tacos or pizza—but low-fat versions should find a permanent place on your weekly menu. One beef-and-cheese taco contains 109 milligrams of calcium, and a slice of vegetarian or cheese pizza contains double that.

Other combination entrées rich in calcium include lasagna, macaroni and cheese, and broccoli quiche.

You can also double or triple the calcium count in many cooked vegetable dishes by preparing them in a cheese sauce. Cooked cauliflower in a cup of cheese sauce, for instance, contains 300 milligrams of calcium.

Tofu and Other Nondairy Foods

Vegetarians have long known about the cooking qualities of tofu, which can be bought in soft cakes that resemble cheese but are made from curdled soy milk. A four-ounce serving of tofu contains 150 milligrams of calcium but only 82 calories, five grams of fat, and no cholesterol. It also soaks up the flavor of any substance it is cooked with. You can use it anywhere you would use cheese or meat—slice it or cube it as a garnish for salads, or add it to casseroles to increase calcium content.

Cook with moderate amounts of molasses; one tablespoon equals 137 milligrams of calcium.

The calcium content of soups, stews, and chicken, fish, or beef stocks that contain bones can be significantly enhanced by adding a little vinegar. The acid in vinegar leaches the calcium from the bones into the soup or stew as it simmers. The result raises the calcium content in a pint of stock equivalent to that of a quart of milk.

Cooking for One

Sometimes people who live alone are tempted not to bother with cooking full meals. They feel they will waste food, because recipes often are designed to serve four to six people, or they simply don't relish putting all that much effort into a meal they will eat alone.

But it is as important for you to prepare balanced, calcium-rich meals whether you are the chef for a dozen people or cooking for yourself.

Do not worry about food going to waste—you can freeze almost any food, so that if you prepare a recipe for four people, you can eat one serving and have three healthy meals waiting for you in your freezer. Any dairy product, including milk and cheese, can be frozen in an airtight bag.

If it seems like a lot of effort to prepare an entrée, remember that you are in effect cooking several meals at once. If you prefer to cook less food at one time, you can halve almost any recipe for four and prepare two servings at a time. And, of course, single-portion servings of milk, cheese, and yogurt do not require you to cook an entire meal.

Storing Dairy Products

Dairy foods can spoil at temperatures at or over about 45 degrees Fahrenheit, at which point bacteria can begin to thrive. You should set your refrigerator between 35 and 40 degrees (marked "Normal" on many refrigerator settings). Do not let dairy products sit on the counter or outside of the refrigerator for extended periods. If milk or another dairy product has been left at a temperature above 45 degrees for more than two hours, it may be spoiled.

Milk containers should be closed tightly, so that they do not absorb flavors or smells of other food inside the refrigerator. Cheese should also be covered tightly and refrigerated. Hard cheese, such as Cheddar, remains edible even after mold develops if an inch around the mold is cut off. Do not eat moldy soft cheese, sour cream, yogurt, or cottage cheese. Carefully check expiration dates on dairy products before using them.

Beware of Calcium Robbers

Finally, in planning your calcium-rich diet, you should beware of the substances on the calcium-inhibitors list. Remember that some substances, such as phytates in high-fiber cereals or unleavened whole-wheat bread, bind calcium so it cannot be absorbed by the body. Don't depend upon a breakfast of a high-fiber bran cereal with milk as a calcium source: you may not absorb the calcium in the milk.

Also keep in mind that excessive salt can cause you to excrete calcium that should be stored in your body. Moderate your use of salt and condiments that are loaded with salt, such as soy sauce and monosodium glutamate (MSG). Artificial salt, now on the market, can help you reduce sodium in cooking. Choose low-sodium bouillon cubes. Discover enticing new flavors to replace saltiness by experimenting with herbs and spices such as oregano, basil, garlic, or sage.

Now that you know how to prepare foods to get the most calcium out of them, chapter eight will tell you how to shop to get the most calcium in your shopping cart.

Shopping for Calcium-Rich Foods

Every food you need for a bone-healthy diet can be found in your local supermarket, and not just in the dairy section. You can find naturally calcium-rich foods in almost every area of the supermarket. The most nutritious and economical choices are usually made by people who plan ahead. Prepare a shopping list that contains high-calcium choices for at least your next few meals. The most important skill you can bring to the supermarket is knowing how to read a food label. Food labels will help you evaluate the nutritional content of food.

The New Food Labels

You'll find a "Nutrition Facts" box on most packaged foods today. Its purpose is to clear up confusion about the nutritional value of products, help you choose healthier diets, and give food companies an incentive to improve the nutritional qualities of their products.

The label provides information about calories, fat,

carbohydrates, sodium, protein, iron, calcium, and vitamins, but it also specifies the amount per serving of saturated fat, cholesterol, dietary fiber, and other nutrients that are of major health concern to shoppers.

You will usually find the "Nutrition Facts" box on the back or side of a package. The information is in large type and must appear on a white or neutral background.

Look first for the serving size at the top of the box. Serving sizes are now set uniformly among similar products so that you can compare competing products reasonably. Serving sizes also now reflect how much people actually eat.

Under the serving size, you'll find how many calories and fat grams a serving contains, and below that the grams of saturated fat, cholesterol, sodium, carbohydrates, and protein. To the right is a column headed "% Daily Values," which, based on a diet of 2,000 calories per day, tells you at a glance whether a food is high or low in fat, cholesterol, sodium, carbohydrates, protein, and fiber in relation to federal dietary recommendations.

The lower portion of the box identifies other key nutrients as a percent of daily value, but not in milligrams. This is where you learn how much calcium one serving contains. To convert the percentage to milligrams, just add a zero to the end of the percentage given (25 percent means 250 milligrams of calcium), since the percentage is based on a calcium RDA of 1,000 milligrams. Read this "% Daily Values" information carefully, however, because here's where the nutrition box falls short in helping shoppers concerned with osteoporosis.

This 1,000-milligram figure, established by the FDA based on the average calcium needs of all ages and populations, may be fine for young men, but may be too low for some people, according to the most recent, reliable recommendations on calcium intake for various populations at risk for osteoporosis. Recall that postmenopausal women on estrogen therapy need 1,200 milligrams of calcium daily, and those not taking estrogen need 1,500 milligrams.

For instance, the Nutrition Facts box on a milk carton claims that one serving (one cup) provides 30 percent of the average person's calcium needs. That translates into 300 milligrams. But 300 milligrams is only 25 percent of 1,200 milligrams—the amount of calcium required by teenage girls, postmenopausal women, pregnant and nursing women, and the elderly of both sexes. Bear in mind this discrepancy when evaluating the calcium content of supermarket foods.

The "% Daily Value" of vitamin D in a food can be found in the same section as that of calcium. This is important for everyone because as we previously discussed, vitamin D is integral to absorbing calcium. The Daily Value for vitamin D is 400 IU (international units). To convert the percentage to an amount, multiply by four. So, if a label states that one serving of a food contains 25 percent of Daily Value, it contains 100 IU of vitamin D.

Health Claims

Another helpful feature of the new label is that the system created uniform definitions for terms that describe a food's nutrient content—such as "light," "low-fat," and "high-fiber"—to ensure that such terms mean the same for any product on which they appear. Fruit-drink labels must also declare the total percentage of juice they contain, so that shoppers will know just how much juice they are getting.

For the first time, products may also carry "health

claims" about the effect of certain nutrients in preventing or treating specific diseases. Currently, the FDA allows eight specific health claims to be carried on some foods. One of them states that calcium-rich foods can reduce the risk of osteoporosis. The other claims are about relationships between:

- fat and greater cancer risk
- saturated fat and cholesterol and greater heart-disease risk
- sodium and greater hypertension risk
- fruits, vegetables, and grains that contain soluble fiber and lower heart-disease risk
- fiber-containing grain products, fruits, and vegetables and lower cancer risk
- fruits and vegetables and lower cancer risk
- folic acid and a lower risk of neural-tube-defect-affected pregnancy

Foods that can claim they are a "high-calcium" source or "rich in calcium" must contain at least 200 milligrams per serving. A "good source" of calcium contains at least 100 milligrams per serving. "More calcium" means the food contains 100 milligrams more calcium than the traditional product.

Similar claims can be made for foods that contain a lot of vitamin D. A food "high in vitamin D" contains 80 IU per serving; a "good source" contains at least 40 IU per serving; food "fortified with vitamin D," at least 40 IU more than an unfortified version.

Ingredients List

Packagers must list ingredients on the food label in descending order by weight. You can usually find the list on the rear or on the side of a package. This list can help the osteoporosis-conscious shopper determine whether nonfat dry milk solids have been added to a food, boosting its calcium content.

Open Dating

Open dating, or freshness dating, is especially important for calcium consumers, since dairy products are perishable. A calendar date is usually stamped on a food package to alert consumers as to its freshness. Dairy products carry a "Sell by" date, which is the last day a product should be sold, assuming that it will then be properly stored at home. To ensure freshness, a good rule of thumb is to treat this date as a "Drink by" deadline. Never buy a product after that date, and try not to eat or drink one after that date. The store, in fact, should pull the food off the shelf after that date.

Now that you know how to read a food label, you are well prepared to shop for calcium-rich and other healthy foods.

Key Words on the New Food Label	
Key Words	What They Mean
Fat	
Fat-free	Less than 0.5 g of fat per serving
Low fat	3 g of fat (or less) per serving
Reduced or less fat	At least 25 percent less per serving than reference food

Saturated Fat

Saturated-fat-free:	Less than 0.5 g, and less than 0.5 g of trans-fatty acids, per serving
Low saturated fat	1 g or less per serving and not more than 15 percent of calories from saturated fatty acids
Reduced or less saturated fat	At least 25 percent less per serving

Cholesterol

Cholesterol-free	Less than 2 mg of cholesterol and 2 g (or less) of saturated fat per serving
Low cholesterol	20 mg or less and 2 g or less of saturated fat per serving and, if the serving is 30 g or less or 2 tablespoons or less, per 50 g of the food
Reduced or less cholesterol	At least 25 percent less than reference food and 2 g or less of saturated fat per serving

The following claims can be used to describe meat, poultry, seafood, and game meats:

Extra-lean	Less than 5 g fat, less than 2 g saturated fat, and less than 95 mg cholesterol per serving and per 100 g

Key Words on the New Food Label *(cont'd.)*

Key Words	What They Mean
Lean	Less than 10 g of fat, 4.5 g of saturated fat, and 95 mg of cholesterol per serving
Light (Lite) Two meanings:	One-third fewer calories or half the fat of the reference food; if the food derives 50 percent or more of its calories from fat, the reduction must be 50 percent of the fat
	or
	a "low-calorie," "low-fat" food whose sodium content has been reduced to 50 percent or less than the reference food; may be used on foods that are not "low-calorie" and "low-fat"
Fiber High fiber	5 g or more per serving
Good source	2.5 g to 4.9 g per serving
More or added fiber	At least 2.5 g more per serving than the reference food

Sugar	
Sugar-free	Less than 0.5 g per serving
No added sugar	No sugar or ingredients that functionally substitute for sugar (such as fruit juice) or ingredients made with added sugars (such as jam)
Reduced sugar	At least 25 percent less sugar than the reference food

Healthy

"Low fat," "low saturated fat," with 60 mg or less cholesterol per serving (or, if raw meat, poultry, or fish, "extra-lean")

At least 10 percent of Daily Value for one or more of vitamins A and C, iron, calcium, protein, and fiber per serving

480 mg or less sodium per serving, and if the serving is 30 g or less or 2 tablespoons or less, per 50 g of the food

(Source: *FDA Consumer*, November 1994)

Shop the Perimeter

The next time you visit your neighborhood supermarket, notice that foods from each category of the Food Guide Pyramid are most likely to be grouped along the perimeter of the store. Although the owners probably had more mercantile concerns in mind when they laid out their goods—ensuring that shoppers peruse the entire store—they created a sensible route that allows health-conscious shoppers to stock up on nutritional foods while largely avoiding the siren call of less healthy enticements beckoning from some of the interior aisles.

Start seeking out calcium-rich foods in the produce section, usually the first section shoppers encounter after walking through the front door. Fill your cart with fresh vegetables and fruits. Low in fat and high in vitamins and fiber, they should make up a major portion of your diet. The American Cancer Society's Five-A-Day campaign calls for eating at least five servings of fruits and vegetables daily to help prevent cancer. Look especially for vegetables that are high in calcium, such as collard greens (360 milligrams per cup), bok choy (250 milligrams per cup), and broccoli (140 milligrams per cup). Look here for tofu, a good calcium source relatively low in fat and high in protein that tastes great in stir-fries or when grilled. Many grocery stores now post nutritional facts in their produce sections for at least the best-selling fruits and vegetables. Use this guide to select the produce richest in calcium.

You won't find many calcium-rich foods at the meat counter, but you can choose smaller portions and lean cuts that will cut down on your fat intake. There are also ways you can use meat to boost your calcium intake. Buy soup bones to make your own stock, which can become calcium-rich if you add a small quantity of vinegar to leach calcium from the bones. Some shellfish are abundant in calcium, especially canned salmon with the bones, which contains 372 milligrams per three ounces. While many lean fresh fish have great nutritional value, it's the bones in canned salmon that provide a great calcium boost. Three ounces of canned pink salmon contains 167 milligrams.

Breads and other goods in the bakery can add smaller amounts of calcium. Remember, grains form the base of the Food Guide Pyramid and should constitute the bulk of your diet, so stock up on healthy grain foods here. Select calcium-fortified bread. Shop for grains that will help you create calcium-rich combination foods, such as pizza or pita bread that you can stuff with mozzarella or another cheese.

Cheese, yogurt, and other milk products can be found on the perimeter in the dairy section, where you will concentrate on stocking up on calcium-rich foods. Remember that some dairy products, although excellent sources of calcium, are also high in fat—a substance you should minimize in your diet. Choose nonfat or low-fat dairy products, or limit the amount of high-fat products.

Steer clear of nondairy creamers, sour cream, butter, and margarine, which you'll find alongside the high-calcium products in most dairy coolers. They contain more saturated fat, fillers, and additives and fewer nutrients, particularly calcium, as an inspection of the label will tell you.

Inside the Perimeter

Food labels such as "calcium-rich" can also flag high-calcium foods along the interior aisles of the super-market. Be cautious in your selections here, however, since many interior aisles contain more highly processed foods and foods containing more fat and sodium. Use the food label to make healthy choices.

Many cereals, for instance, have been fortified with calcium and vitamin D along with other vitamins and minerals. High-fiber cereals are not the best choice, since fiber, as discussed in chapter five, may interfere with calcium absorption. Another poor choice is cereals high in sugar. Read the food label to make the best selection, to optimize calcium intake, and minimize sugar and/or fat intake.

Some snack foods are fortified with calcium. One

example is chewy chocolate-chip-flavored Carnation Breakfast Bars: one bar provides half the "% Daily Value" for calcium (500 milligrams). Instant breakfast drinks also provide a quick and easy breakfast or snack. The vanilla Carnation Instant Breakfast provides 500 milligrams of calcium after you add one cup of skim milk.

Pancake mixes offer another calcium-rich breakfast. Buttermilk-pancake mixes contain more than double the calcium of regular mixes, but they also contain three times the fat. An alternative is to add nonfat dry milk to your regular brand of pancake mix. You can find nonfat dry milk solids and nonfat buttermilk in the baking section, along with evaporated skim milk. All of these products can help you boost calcium content in meals that you cook. Other mixes that offer high calcium include macaroni and cheese, burrito or taco kits (you add fresh cheese), broccoli in cheese sauce, and instant pudding. Read the labels and you'll find even more, but keep track of fat, sodium, and additives.

The freezer section offers another wealth of calcium-rich foods, although many frozen entrées are laden with sodium and/or fat. But you can find healthy choices. If you are pushed for time, frozen convenience dinners are an excellent way to keep up with your calcium needs (see the accompanying table).

Frozen milk products offer a tasty way to take in some calcium. Supermarkets stock a wide range of low-fat frozen-yogurt treats as well as the richer ice cream. Some ice creams are lower in fat than others. Changes in governmental standards of identity (federal regulations on how a company can label a food) now permit companies to label as ice cream low-fat foods that formerly were known as ice milk or a dairy dessert because of their lower fat content.

Calcium Content of Some Frozen Foods

Food	Calories	% Daily Value Total Fat	% Daily Value Sodium	% Daily Value Calcium
Tombstone Pepperoni Pizza ⅕ pizza (one slice)	340	18	31	25
Tombstone for One Vegetarian Pizza	360	15	30	30
Healthy Choice Garden Potato Casserole (9.5 oz.)	200	6	22	10
Healthy Choice Chicken Parmigiana	300	3	21	10
Stouffer's Four Cheese Lasagna (10 oz.)	580	61	34	25
Michelina's Macaroni & Cheese (9 oz.)	370	23	31	25
Weight Watchers Tuna Noodle Casserole (11.5 oz.)	240	11	24	15
Weight Watchers Chicken Fettucini (8.25 oz.)	280	14	25	20
Michelina's Bean & Cheese Enchiladas (10.5 oz.)	420	24	48	40
The Budget Gourmet Wide Ribbon Pasta with Ricotta and Chunky Tomato Sauce (10.25 oz.)	420	34	26	30
The Budget Gourmet Four Cheese Rice, Pasta and Chicken (10.5 oz.)	330	20	35	20

Calcium Content of Some Frozen Foods (cont'd.)				
Food	Calories	% Daily Value Total Fat	% Daily Value Sodium	% Daily Value Calcium
Birds Eye Broccoli with Cheese Sauce (4 oz.)	70	5	18	10
Pictsweet Cut Okra (6 oz.)	25	0	1	6
Hungry Jack Microwave Buttermilk Pancakes (3 pancakes)	240	6	24	8
Lean Pockets Chicken Parmesan (1 sandwich)	260	12	26	20
Fiesta Bagel Bites Nacho Flavor (4 bagels)	200	11	26	15
Steak-umm Microwave Cheesesteak to Go (5.6 oz.)	480	40	30	25

Supermarkets Versus Specialty Stores

Supermarkets have responded to the public interest in healthier foods by expanding their natural-foods selections so that most are quite competitive with health-food stores—and at lower prices. You can find a great variety of so-called health foods—ranging from sesame tahini to fruit-sweetened jam to couscous—at virtually any super-market.

That applies to the dairy section as well. In addition to traditional dairy products, shoppers seeking rich cal-cium sources can find acidophilus milk (for the lactose-intolerant), buttermilk, and yogurt with active cultures in the dairy cooler.

Products sold at health-food stores or other alter-native-food stores are almost always more expensive than those in the supermarket. Often, they are no more nutritious than those you can buy in a supermarket. Health-food stores do offer excellent organic fruits and vegetables. "Organically grown" means that neither the produce nor the ground in which it grew has been treated by chemicals, fertilizers, or pesticides. Only manure or compost has been used as fertilizer. It is important to wash organically grown foods well to rid them of any fecal matter, which can cause health prob-lems of its own.

In addition to organically grown foods, health-food stores usually sell an impressive selection of grains, rice, and other dry goods in bulk, which can hold down their price. You'll find as many dairy foods in a health-food store as in a supermarket, if not more.

One kind of milk you will not find in a supermarket but may in an alternative health-food store is raw milk. Raw milk has not been pasteurized (heated) to kill germs that can cause disease. Some people argue that raw milk is healthier than pasteurized milk because the heating process kills nutrients. But heating cannot destroy minerals (such as calcium), and drinking unpasteurized milk poses health risks. The danger of acquiring a fatal bacterial infection such as salmonella from raw milk or cheese made from it is greater for the elderly, children, and the chronically ill. At least 25 states ban raw milk. Pasteurized milk is a safer and equally calcium-rich choice.

Health-food stores may offer some excellent calcium supplements, but again, stay away from any that contain dolomite or bone meal, which may contain excessive amounts of lead or other toxins. Read the ingredients label.

Diet Deception and Quackery

Stricter federal regulations have closed loopholes that allowed packagers to make misleading claims about foods on their labels. With the exception of the labels described earlier in this chapter, food manufacturers can make no claim about the relationship between a food and a disease. Labels can say that a high-calcium diet is associated with a lower risk for osteoporosis only because scientific research strongly supports that statement.

Now that you know how to prepare and buy food to maximize its calcium content, chapter nine will give you recipes for cooking delicious, calcium-rich meals.

Calcium-Rich Recipes

A
t the Stedman Center we believe that for any diet regimen to work, it must be simple and tasty. The following recipes collected by nutritionists at the Stedman Center fill that bill and also provide you with plenty of crucial calcium.

One of the most pleasant surprises about embarking on a calcium-rich diet is that cooking with calcium is simple and delicious. The recipes require no exotic ingredients to boost your calcium intake, and the ingredients that fill recipes with calcium are as close as your nearest dairy counter. Better yet, these calcium-rich recipes taste great.

Remember, cooking from scratch is one way to ensure that the foods you eat contain maximum calcium and minimum fat. You can add more nonfat dairy products and less butter or fat to your soups, casseroles, and other foods than manufacturers do.

All of the recipes can be adapted to cooking for one. You can reduce the ingredients proportionately or freeze leftovers (see chapter seven).

The recipes appear under the following category headings: Breakfast Dishes; Pasta Entrées; Other Lunch and Dinner Entrées; Salad, Vegetable, and Side Dishes; Soups; Bread and Muffins; Sauce, Dressing, and Dip Blends; and Snacks and Desserts.

Breakfast
Dishes

Blueberry Pancakes

1½	cups buttermilk
1	egg
1½	cups all-purpose flour (or 1 cup all-purpose + ½ cup whole-wheat flour)
½	teaspoon baking soda
1	teaspoon baking powder
1	tablespoon sugar
3	tablespoons nonfat dry milk powder
1	cup blueberries
2	tablespoons water (optional)
	nonstick spray

Combine wet and dry, leaving mixture somewhat lumpy. Stir in blueberries (or drop a few onto each pancake while cooking). If batter is too dry, add optional water. Cook in a nonstick skillet sprayed with nonstick spray, measuring two ounces of batter per pancake. Serve immediately.

Yield: 10 pancakes

Calories per pancake: 106
Calcium: 72 mg
Fat: 1 g
Sodium: 127 mg

French Toast

½	cup water
⅓	cup nonfat dry milk powder
4	egg whites
1	teaspoon sugar
¼	teaspoon vanilla extract
	sprinkle of cinnamon
6	slices whole-wheat bread
	nonstick spray

Combine water and nonfat dry milk in pie plate. Stir in egg whites, sugar, vanilla, and cinnamon. Dip both sides of bread in egg mixture. Brown in a nonstick pan sprayed with nonstick spray. Serve hot.

Yield: 3 servings (2 slices each)

Calories per serving: 273
Calcium: 135 mg
Fat: 0 g
Sodium: 470 mg

Apricot Almond Granola

4	cups old-fashioned rolled oats
1	cup nonfat dry milk powder
1	cup chopped dried apricots
½	cup toasted wheat germ
½	cup slivered almonds
2	teaspoons ground cinnamon
1¼	cups firmly packed brown sugar
¼	cup water
¾	cup canola oil
2	teaspoons vanilla extract

Combine oats, nonfat dry milk, apricots, wheat germ, almonds, and cinnamon in a large bowl. Heat sugar and water to a full boil and let cool slightly. Stir in oil and vanilla. Stir into oat mixture until all is moistened. Spread on ungreased 15½-by-10½-by-1-inch jelly-roll pan. Bake in very slow oven (200°F.) for 2–2½ hours, or until dry, stirring every 30 minutes. Let cool. Can be stored in an airtight container in a cool, dry place for one month. Serve as a dry snack, or with milk for breakfast.

Yield: 18 servings (½ cup each)

Calories per serving: 263
Calcium: 81 mg
Fat: 12 g
Sodium: 27 mg

Morning Fruit Shake

1   cup skim milk
1   cup sliced ripe banana
3   tablespoons frozen orange-juice concentrate
½   teaspoon pure vanilla extract

In the container of an electric blender, place milk, banana, orange juice, and vanilla extract. Cover and whirl until smooth. Serve at once.

Yield: 2 servings (7 ounces each)

Calories per serving: 133
Calcium: 161 mg
Fat: 1 g
Sodium: 64 mg

Morning Fruit Shake with Yogurt

1	cup nonfat plain yogurt
½	cup skim milk
2	tablespoons honey
2	teaspoons pure vanilla extract
1	cup sliced fruit, such as bananas, strawberries, peaches, pears, pineapple

In the container of an electric blender, place yogurt, milk, honey, vanilla extract, and fruit. Cover and whirl until smooth. Pour into 2 large glasses. Serve immediately.

Yield: 2 servings (8 ounces each)

Calories per serving: 217
Calcium: 306 mg
Fat: 1 g
Sodium: 120 mg

Banana Smoothie

¾ cup skim milk
2 tablespoons nonfat dry milk powder
½ banana
3 packets Equal®
  mint sprig (optional garnish)
  fruit (optional garnish)

Combine skim milk, nonfat dry milk, banana, and Equal® in a blender. Process on high speed until smooth. Garnish with sprig of mint and fresh fruit if desired.

Variation: Any fruit or combination of fruits may be substituted for banana.

Yield: 1 serving (8 ounces)

Calories per serving: 160
Calcium: 333 mg
Fat: 1 g
Sodium: 154 mg

Note: If banana is frozen ahead of time, it makes a thicker shake when blended.

Pasta Entrées

Adam's Fettuccine

A delicious low-fat version of fettuccine Alfredo.

8	ounces fettuccine or linguine
1	tablespoon olive oil
¾	cup evaporated skim milk
⅓	cup + 4 teaspoons grated Parmesan cheese
¼	cup sliced green onion
2	tablespoons snipped fresh basil or ½ teaspoon dried basil, crushed
¼	teaspoon finely shredded lemon peel
¼	teaspoon garlic powder
⅛	teaspoon ground black pepper

Cook pasta according to package directions. Drain, then immediately return to pan. Add oil and toss to coat. Add the milk, the ⅓ cup cheese, and the onion, basil, lemon peel, garlic powder, and pepper. Cook over medium-high heat until bubbly, stirring constantly. Top with 4 teaspoons cheese.

Yield: 4 servings (1 cup each)

Calories per serving: 344
Calcium: 343 mg
Fat: 9 g
Sodium: 325 mg

Cheesy Macaroni

This is a reduced-fat recipe using four cheeses—cottage, mozzarella, Cheddar, and Parmesan.

1	8-ounce package uncooked elbow macaroni
1½	cups low-fat (1 percent) cottage cheese
1	cup shredded part-skim mozzarella cheese
2	cups shredded low-fat Cheddar cheese
2	egg whites
¾	cup skim milk
2	tablespoons finely chopped onion
1	teaspoon Worcestershire sauce
½	teaspoon dry mustard
⅛	teaspoon white pepper (optional) paprika
1	teaspoon Parmesan cheese

Heat oven to moderate (325°–350°F). Cook macaroni according to package directions and drain. Combine cottage, mozzarella, and Cheddar cheeses, egg whites, milk, onion, Worcestershire sauce, dry mustard, and pepper in a large bowl. Mix until blended, and fold in macaroni. Spoon mixture into a 2½-quart casserole dish. Sprinkle with paprika and Parmesan cheese. Bake for 20–30 minutes, or until bubbly.

Yield: 7 servings

Calories per serving: 231
Calcium: 413 mg
Fat: 9 g
Sodium: 418 mg

Note: This dish may be frozen prior to baking. When ready to use, thaw and bake as above.

Vegetarian Lasagna

1	pound lasagna noodles
1	teaspoon olive oil
1½	cups diced onion
2	pounds mushrooms, sliced
1	teaspoon dried rosemary
1	teaspoon dried oregano
1	pound zucchini, thinly sliced
⅓	pound part-skim ricotta cheese
3	egg whites
⅓	pound part-skim mozzarella cheese, grated
3	cups low-fat tomato spaghetti sauce
½	cup chopped fresh parsley
2	tablespoons grated Parmesan cheese

Cook lasagna noodles al dente, drain, and set aside in cool water. Preheat oven to 350°F. Heat the olive oil in a skillet and sauté the onion, mushrooms, rosemary, and oregano. Continue to cook until liquid evaporates. Add zucchini and cook until soft. Set vegetable mixture aside in a colander to drain and cool.

Mix ricotta, egg whites, and grated mozzarella (reserving 3 tablespoons for topping). Assemble lasagna in an 8-by-11-by-12-inch casserole dish. Place 1 cup sauce on bottom of casserole, then cover with a layer of lasagna noodles. Spread ½ of vegetable mixture over noodles, followed by ½ of cheese mixture and another layer of noodles. Repeat the layering process and cover the top layer of noodles with a thin layer of sauce. Sprinkle the parsley and Parmesan and reserved mozzarella over the casserole and bake uncovered for 30–40 minutes. To serve, remove lasagna from the oven and allow it to set for 10 minutes before cutting.

Yield: 12 servings

Calories per serving: 218
Calcium: 159 mg
Fat: 4 g
Sodium: 472 mg

Tomato and Pepper Ziti

8	ounces ziti, or other pasta of choice
1	teaspoon olive oil
2	cloves garlic, chopped
1	bag frozen bell peppers, or 2 cups julienne-sliced fresh bell peppers (red, green, yellow)
1	cup chopped tomatoes, fresh or canned
1	teaspoon dried basil
⅛	teaspoon ground black pepper
6	ounces part-skim mozzarella cheese
1	tablespoon grated Parmesan cheese

Cook pasta according to package directions, drain, and set aside. In sauté pan, heat olive oil. Add garlic and sauté. Add peppers and tomatoes and sauté. Add basil, black pepper, and mozzarella. Mix well until thoroughly heated. Serve over cooked pasta. Top with freshly grated Parmesan cheese.

Yield: 4 servings

Calories per serving: 319
Calcium: 353 mg
Fat: 10 g
Sodium: 257 mg

Pasta, Peas, and Onions

12	ounces spaghetti
5	cups chopped onion
1½	cups frozen peas, cooked
½	cup grated Parmesan cheese
	salt and ground black pepper to taste
	nonstick spray

Bring large pot of (unsalted) water to boil and add pasta. Cook until al dente, stirring often, about 12 minutes or per package directions. Meanwhile, spray heavy large skillet with nonstick spray and heat over medium heat. Add chopped onion and sauté until golden, about 5 minutes. Add peas and sauté until tender, about 3 minutes. When pasta is done, drain it and return it to pot. Add onion mixture and grated cheese. Toss to combine. Transfer pasta to bowl.

Yield: 5 servings (½ cup each)

Calories per serving: 246
Calcium: 204 mg
Fat: 4 g
Sodium: 258 mg

Pasta with Spinach

2   cups cooked (approximately 8 ounces) pasta, such as spaghetti

12   ounces spaghetti sauce (Classico spicy red pepper works well)

1   cup spinach (frozen or fresh)

1   cup low-fat (1 percent) or nonfat cottage cheese

¼   cup grated Parmesan cheese

Cook the pasta until al dente. Heat the spaghetti sauce until hot. Cook the spinach (microwave works great). Layer the pasta, then spinach, then cottage cheese on the serving plate. Pour the hot spaghetti sauce over top of it and sprinkle with the Parmesan cheese. This makes a great substitute for spinach lasagna without all the work. The hot spaghetti sauce melts the cheese to make it rich and creamy-tasting!

Yield: 4 servings

Calories per serving: 269
Calcium: 202 mg
Fat: 7 g
Sodium: 787 mg

Tuna Bake

12	ounces shells or other shaped pasta, uncooked
2	teaspoons olive oil
1½	cups diced celery
1	cup sliced water chestnuts, drained and rinsed
2	cups diced green bell pepper (fresh or frozen)
1	onion, diced
1	15-ounce can stewed tomatoes
2	cloves garlic, minced
½	cup skim milk
2	tablespoons all-purpose flour
6	ounces Swiss cheese, shredded
1	tablespoon dried dill weed
½	teaspoon ground black pepper
¼	teaspoon cayenne pepper
1	6-ounce can water-packed tuna, drained nonstick spray
½	cup Parmesan cheese

Cook pasta and set aside. Preheat oven to 350°F. Sauté celery, water chestnuts, peppers, onions, tomatoes, and garlic in olive oil. Add milk, flour, and Swiss cheese. Simmer until sauce thickens. Stir in dill, black pepper, cayenne pepper, and tuna. Remove from heat and mix in cooked pasta. Prepare an 8-cup casserole dish with nonstick spray. Pour pasta mixture in and sprinkle with Parmesan cheese. Bake 35–45 minutes.

Yield: 8 servings (1 cup each)

Calories per serving: 335   Fat: 9 g
Calcium: 346 mg   Sodium: 267 mg

Shrimp Scampi

¾ cup carrots cut on the bias
¾ cup snow peas
2 cloves garlic, minced
2 cups chicken stock
2 tablespoons lemon juice
2 tablespoons cornstarch
3 tablespoons buttermilk
1½ tablespoons grated Parmesan
pinch of salt (optional)
⅛ teaspoon white pepper
2 tablespoons chopped fresh parsley
8 ounces linguine
1 pound shrimp
1 lemon, cut in 6 wedges

Steam carrots for 2 minutes, or until al dente, and set aside. Steam the snow peas for 30 seconds and set aside. Make sauce by combining the garlic, stock, and lemon juice. Bring to a boil. Dissolve the cornstarch in the buttermilk and add to the broth. Add Parmesan cheese, salt, pepper, and 1 tablespoon of the chopped parsley, then simmer until slightly thickened. Cook linguine until al dente, drain, and add to sauce. Steam shrimp for approximately 3 minutes. Add vegetables to sauce, then place pasta, sauce, and vegetable combination on plate, top with shrimp, and garnish with remaining chopped parsley and the lemon.

Yield: 6 servings

Calories per serving: 166   Fat: 2 g
Calcium: 93 mg   Sodium: 259 mg

Other Lunch and Dinner Entrées

Creamy Dijon Chicken and Broccoli

8   ounces chicken breast, diced
2   cups brown rice (or instant or Minute Rice)
1   cup pasta, such as bowties or macaroni
2   cups chopped broccoli (fresh or frozen)
1   10½-ounce can low-fat cream of mushroom, celery, or broccoli soup
1½ teaspoons Dijon mustard
½   cup skim milk
1   cup canned mushrooms, drained
    ground black pepper to taste
    bread crumbs or Parmesan cheese for topping (optional)

Cook chicken breast and set aside (steam in microwave, boil, use leftovers—or leave this ingredient out and make the dish vegetarian-style). Cook rice and pasta according to package directions or just use leftover rice or pasta. Put frozen broccoli in pan and cook on medium-low heat with about ¼ to ⅓ cup water, or microwave. If your broccoli is fresh, then you can just add it when you mix all of the ingredients.

In a saucepan large enough to hold all the ingredients, heat the can of soup, Dijon mustard, and milk. Add water to thin to desired consistency. Stir in cooked rice and pasta. Add broccoli, mushrooms, chicken, if using, and pepper to taste. Cook until heated through. You can top it with bread crumbs and/or Parmesan cheese if you desire.

Yield: 8 servings

Calories per serving: 168
Calcium: 52 mg
Fat: 4 g
Sodium: 314 mg

Broccoli Quiche

Crust:

4	cups cooked brown rice
2	cloves garlic, minced
4	egg whites
	nonstick spray

Filling:

6	cups fresh broccoli chopped into ½-inch pieces
1	teaspoon olive oil
3	green onions, sliced
3	cloves garlic, minced
1½	cups evaporated skim milk
1	teaspoon dried basil
½	teaspoon dried thyme
	several dashes cayenne pepper
4	egg whites, lightly beaten
⅓	cup + 1 tablespoon Parmesan cheese
2	small tomatoes, sliced

Preheat oven to 375°F. Mix together cooked brown rice, garlic, and 4 egg whites in medium-sized bowl. Lightly spray a 9-by-12-inch pan with nonstick spray. Spoon in rice mixture, lining bottom and sides with rice, pressing rice into place slightly with spoon. Meanwhile, cook broccoli until tender-crisp by placing a steamer basket over 1 inch of water and cooking covered about 5 minutes. Heat oil in a large nonstick skillet over medium-high heat. Add green onions and garlic. Sauté 3 minutes. Remove pan from heat. Add steamed broccoli, evaporated skim milk, basil, thyme, cayenne pepper, 4 egg whites lightly beaten, and ⅓ cup Parmesan cheese. Spoon mixture evenly over rice in pan. Arrange tomato slices evenly over quiche. Sprinkle each tomato slice with Parmesan cheese, using 1 tablespoon total. Bake for 30 minutes.

Yield: 14 servings

Calories per serving: 122
Calcium: 142 mg
Fat: 2 g
Sodium: 120 mg

Stuffed Peppers

2	cups diced onion
1¼	cups diced bell pepper
1¾	cups sliced mushrooms
2	cloves garlic, minced
⅓	cup low-fat (1 percent) cottage cheese
3	tablespoons tomato paste
1	cup cooked white rice
2	tablespoons grated Parmesan cheese
¼	teaspoon dried basil
¼	teaspoon dried oregano
⅛	teaspoon ground black pepper
3	green bell peppers, halved lengthwise and seeded

Preheat oven to 350°F. To make filling, sweat onion, diced bell pepper, mushrooms, and garlic in a covered skillet with a little water. Combine softened vegetables with remaining ingredients except pepper halves. Stuff pepper halves, place in a baking dish, and bake for 1 hour, or until peppers are soft.

Yield: 6 servings

Calories per serving: 110
Calcium: 58 mg
Fat: 1 g
Sodium: 151 mg

Baked Cheese
and Ham Hero

1   loaf (8 ounces) Italian bread
4   ounces part-skim mozzarella cheese
1   cup shredded low-fat sharp Cheddar
    cheese
2   ounces boiled ham, sliced
1   medium-sized ripe tomato, thinly sliced
½   teaspoon Italian seasoning, crushed

Preheat oven to 350°F. Slice bread in half lengthwise. On bottom half, place both cheeses, ham, and tomato. Sprinkle with Italian seasoning. Cover with top half of loaf. Place in the center of a 12-inch length of aluminum foil. Bring sides of foil around loaf, leaving uncovered a half-inch-wide strip along the top of the bread (this results in a crisp crust). Gently press foil around bread. Bake until it's hot and cheese is melted, about 25 minutes. Cut into 5 portions. Serve hot.

Yield: 5 servings

Calories per serving: 229
Calcium: 280 mg
Fat: 10 g
Sodium: 556 mg

Super Easy Vegetable Crepes

½   onion, chopped
1   tablespoon minced garlic (from jar)
    any vegetables that look good in the
    grocery store's salad bar and that
    you don't have to clean or cut
1   10½-ounce Healthy Request (or other
    low-sodium, low-fat brand) cream of
    mushroom or cream of broccoli soup
¾   cup skim milk
8   prepared crepes (check the fruit
    section of a good grocery store)

This is easier than it sounds and is sure to impress. Sauté onion and garlic for about 5 minutes or less in something. (You can use 1 tablespoon butter/margarine/oil, or you can substitute ¼–⅓ cup or so of water, beer, fruit juice, or wine—if it looks dry, just add more.) Add vegetables from the salad-bar line (carrots, zucchini, summer squash, mushrooms, peas, spinach—anything) or add frozen vegetables (again, anything you like). Let cook about 5–7 minutes. Open soup can. Add ¾ cup of skim milk to soup concentrate and pour into the cooking veggies, reserving ½ cup to top crepes. Let it cook some more, until it is hot and as done as you like it. Open crepes, pull one out, and fill it with the vegetable-and-sauce mixture (about ⅓ cup is all it takes). Pour a little of the reserved sauce over the top of the crepe. One 9-inch saucepan of veggies will fill 8–10 crepes. A wonderful one-pan dish.

Yield: 8 servings

Calories per serving: 128
Calcium: 85 mg
Fat: 3 g
Sodium: 317 mg

Crustless Italian Vegetable and Cheese Pie

½   cup each thinly sliced carrot, zucchini, celery, and onion
8   egg whites
1   15-ounce package low-fat ricotta cheese
½   teaspoon dried basil, crushed
    pinch ground black pepper
1   cup (4 ounces) diced part-skim mozzarella cheese
    nonstick spray

Preheat oven to 350°F. In a large skillet, bring 1 inch water to a boil. Add carrot, zucchini, celery, and onion. Simmer, covered, until almost tender, about 5 minutes. Drain and set aside. In a large bowl, beat egg whites. Add ricotta cheese, basil, and black pepper and mix well. Stir in mozzarella cheese and ¾ of the reserved vegetables. Pour into quiche dish sprayed with nonstick spray. Top with remaining vegetables. Bake until a knife inserted in the center comes out clean.

Yield: 6 servings

Calories per serving: 174
Calcium: 324 mg
Fat: 9 g
Sodium: 254 mg

Barbecue Chicken Pita Pizza

3	ounces raw chicken breast, trimmed
1½	tablespoons barbecue sauce
1	2-ounce pita bread
¼	cup chopped onion
½	cup sliced mushrooms
¼	cup chopped green bell pepper
2	ounces part-skim mozzarella cheese

Steam, boil, or microwave chicken breast until done. Leftover chicken from the grill or stir-fried chicken is also great and makes preparation even quicker.

Preheat oven to 450°F. Spread barbecue sauce on the unopened pita. Sauté onions, mushrooms, and peppers in nonstick pan. Spread chicken, vegetables, and cheese on pita. Bake for 7–10 minutes.

This recipe also works great using a ready-made crust.

Yield: 1 personal pizza

Calories per serving: 448
Calcium: 441 mg
Fat: 12 g
Sodium: 851 mg

Bean Burrito

¼	teaspoon olive oil
2	tablespoons diced onion
⅛	cup diced green bell pepper
¼	cup canned nonfat refried beans
1	tortilla shell
½	ounce Cheddar cheese
1	tablespoon nonfat plain yogurt
⅛	cup chopped lettuce
1	tablespoon diced tomato
1	tablespoon salsa

Heat oil in a skillet and sauté onion and pepper over medium-high heat. Lower to medium heat and add beans. Dilute with water as needed so that you can stir without sticking. Simmer until beans are smooth and creamy. Heat tortilla shell. Fill with beans, cheese, yogurt, lettuce, tomato, and salsa.

Yield: 1 burrito

Calories per serving: 225
Calcium: 210 mg
Fat: 8 g
Sodium: 384 mg

Baked Catfish

⅓   cup all-purpose flour
⅓   cup bread crumbs
1½   teaspoons paprika
     pinch of salt (optional)
⅛   teaspoon ground black pepper
2   tablespoons grated Parmesan cheese
2   pounds catfish fillets
¾   cup nonfat plain yogurt
     nonstick spray

Preheat oven to 450°F. Mix flour, bread crumbs, paprika, salt, pepper, and cheese. Divide fish into six pieces. Coat catfish in yogurt, then dredge in breading mix. Spray two baking sheets with nonstick spray and bake the catfish for 10 minutes, or until done.

Yield: 6 servings

Calories per serving: 235
Calcium: 141 mg
Fat: 8 g
Sodium: 160 mg

Chili Baked Chicken and Rice

Rice cooked in milk gives this unusual chicken meal-in-a-dish a calcium bonus.

	nonstick spray
1	cup uncooked rice
½	cup sliced green onions
3	cups skim milk
⅛	teaspoon ground black pepper
1	teaspoon chili powder
6	chicken breast halves, skinned and boned (about 30 ounces)

Preheat oven to 350°F. Spray a 12-by-9-by-2-inch casserole dish with nonstick spray. Add rice and green onions. Combine milk and black pepper and pour over rice. Rub chili powder into all sides of chicken. Arrange chicken over rice. Bake, uncovered, gently stirring rice occasionally, until chicken is cooked through and crisp, about 55 minutes. Stir rice and set aside for 5 minutes, till milk is absorbed, before serving.

Yield: 6 servings (½ chicken breast and ½ cup rice each)

Calories per serving: 316
Calcium: 183 mg
Fat: 6 g
Sodium: 162 mg

Salad, Vegetable, and Side Dishes

Cucumber Salad

4	large cucumbers
1	cup nonfat plain yogurt
2	tablespoons cider vinegar
1	tablespoon Dijon mustard
½	cup sliced red onion (¼-inch slices)
¼	cup thinly sliced green onions
¼	cup finely diced red bell pepper
¼	teaspoon (or less) finely ground black pepper

Peel cucumbers and cut in half lengthwise. Remove seeds, then cut into ¼-inch slices (they'll be shaped like half-moons). In a large bowl, combine yogurt, vinegar, and mustard. Add cucumbers, onion, green onion, and bell pepper. Mix well and add pepper.

Yield: 6 servings (scant ½ cup each)

Calories per serving: 52
Calcium: 98 mg
Fat: 1 g
Sodium: 63 mg

Rebaked Stuffed Potatoes

2	medium baking potatoes
3	tablespoons nonfat plain yogurt
½	cup low-fat (1-percent) cottage cheese
¾	cup shredded part-skim mozzarella cheese
¼	cup skim milk (approximately)
½	teaspoon dried dill weed
1	teaspoon dry mustard
	paprika
1	teaspoon grated Parmesan cheese

Bake potatoes in 400°F. oven for 1 hour, or until done. When cool enough to handle, slice lengthwise and scoop out inside, leaving skins intact. In a bowl, mash warm potatoes with yogurt, cottage cheese, ½ cup of the mozzarella cheese, and milk. Add the dill weed and dry mustard and mix well. Stuff the skins with this mixture. Top with remaining ¼ cup mozzarella cheese, paprika, and Parmesan cheese. Rebake potatoes for approximately 20 minutes. May be frozen.

Yield: 4 servings (½ potato each)

Calories per serving: 164
Calcium: 210 mg
Fat: 4 g
Sodium: 261 mg

Mashed Potatoes

3½	pounds potatoes, peeled and diced
4	cups buttermilk
½	cup nonfat dry milk powder
1	tablespoon salt

Place potatoes in a pot and cover with water, bring to a boil, and simmer until soft. Drain, reserve some of the cooking liquid, and mash. Dissolve milk powder in buttermilk. Add buttermilk mixture, salt, and cooking liquid as needed.

Yield: 12 servings (¾ cup each)

Calories per serving: 157
Calcium: 143 mg
Fat: 1 g
Sodium: 286 mg

Crispy Potato Scallop

nonstick spray
4 cups (about 2 pounds) peeled and thinly sliced potatoes
1 cup thinly sliced onions
¼ cup reduced-calorie margarine
½ cup Italian-style bread crumbs
2 cups skim milk

Preheat oven to 325°F. Spray a shallow 2-quart casserole dish with nonstick spray and set aside. Layer half the potatoes and half the onions in casserole. Dot with half the margarine and half the bread crumbs. Repeat layering with remaining onions, potatoes, margarine, and bread crumbs. Pour skim milk over all. Cover and bake for 45 minutes. Uncover and bake until potatoes are tender and almost all of the liquid is absorbed, about 50 minutes longer.

Yield: 8 servings (½ cup each)

Calories per serving: 175
Calcium: 97 mg
Fat: 3 g
Sodium: 149 mg

Soups

Vegetable Cheddar Chowder

2	tablespoons reduced-calorie margarine
1	cup diced zucchini
½	cup chopped onion
½	cup diced green bell pepper
¼	cup thinly sliced carrot
2	tablespoons all-purpose flour
3	cups skim milk
1	cup shredded low-fat Cheddar cheese
¹⁄₁₆	teaspoon ground black pepper

In a medium saucepan, melt margarine. Add zucchini, onion, green pepper, and carrot and sauté until onion is tender, about 5 minutes. Stir in flour; cook and stir for 1 minute. Gradually stir in milk; cook and stir until mixture boils and thickens. Blend in Cheddar cheese and black pepper; heat and stir just until cheese melts. Serve hot.

Yield: 4 servings (7 ounces each)

Calories per serving: 178
Calcium: 444 mg
Fat: 8 g
Sodium: 252 mg

Broccoli–Swiss Cheese Soup

3½   cups skim milk
½   cup evaporated skim milk
1½   teaspoons cornstarch
¼   teaspoon ground black pepper
     dash of hot sauce
¼   teaspoon dry mustard
1   cup shredded low-fat Swiss cheese
1   10-ounce package frozen chopped
     broccoli, thawed and drained
¼   teaspoon butter substitute (such as Molly
     McButter or Butter Buds)
     chopped chives (optional)
     carrot curls (optional)

Combine skim milk, evaporated milk, cornstarch, pepper, hot sauce, and mustard in a large saucepan and mix well. Cook over medium heat, stirring constantly, until smooth and thickened. Add ½ cup of the cheese and stir until cheese melts. Add broccoli and butter substitute, then cook until thoroughly heated. Ladle into 3 bowls and sprinkle with remaining ½ cup cheese. Garnish with chives and carrot, if desired.

Yield: 3 servings (9 ounces each)

Calories per serving: 294
Calcium: 525 mg
Fat: 10 g
Sodium: 266 mg

Zucchini Yogurt Soup

3	cups chopped onion
4	cups chopped zucchini
1	tablespoon olive oil
6	cups chicken broth, canned, low-sodium
½	teaspoon ground black pepper
¼	cup chopped fresh dill, plus extra for garnish
1	cup low-fat plain yogurt, plus extra for garnish

Coarsely chop onion and zucchini and sauté in olive oil in heavy-bottomed soup pot. When onion is translucent, add chicken broth. Bring to a boil, then simmer for approximately 45 minutes. Remove from heat; add pepper and dill. When cool, purée in blender, then whisk in yogurt. Serve garnished with chopped dill and a dollop of yogurt.

Yield: 10 servings (1 cup each)

Calories per serving: 79
Calcium: 85 mg
Fat: 3 g
Sodium: 487 mg

Bread and Muffins

Corn Bread

nonstick spray
1½ cups cornmeal
½   cup all-purpose flour
1   tablespoon baking powder
½   teaspoon baking soda
1⅓ cups buttermilk
2   tablespoons apple-juice concentrate
2   egg whites

Heat oven to 425°F. Spray 8-inch pan with nonstick spray. Mix cornmeal, flour, baking powder, and baking soda and set aside. Mix buttermilk and apple juice. In mixer, beat egg whites until stiff. Add cornmeal mixture to buttermilk mixture, and mix with a fork. Fold in egg whites. Pour into prepared pan and bake immediately for 20 minutes, or until brown

Yield: 12 servings

Calories per serving: 93
Calcium: 49 mg
Fat: 8 g
Sodium: 160 mg

Lemon Muffins

1¾	cups all-purpose flour
¾	cup sugar
1	teaspoon baking soda
¼	teaspoon salt
1	cup nonfat plain yogurt
3	tablespoons margarine
1	egg
1	tablespoon fresh lemon juice
1	tablespoon grated lemon zest
¼	teaspoon lemon extract
	nonstick spray

Preheat oven to 350°F. In separate bowls, combine dry and wet ingredients. Mix dry and wet ingredients together until just incorporated. Spray muffin tin with nonstick spray. Bake about 12 minutes.

Yield: 12 muffins (1 per serving)

Calories per serving: 159
Calcium: 39 mg
Fat: 4 g
Sodium: 176 mg

Sauce, Dressing, and Dip Blends

Creamy Dill Sauce

	nonstick spray
1	tablespoon minced onion
1	tablespoon cornstarch
½	teaspoon dried dill weed
	pinch of ground black pepper
1	cup skim milk
½	cup nonfat plain yogurt

Spray a saucepan with nonstick spray and sauté onion until tender. In a small bowl, combine cornstarch, dill, black pepper, and milk. Stir into saucepan. Bring to a boil. Cook and stir over medium heat until thickened, about 1 minute. Remove from heat and stir in yogurt. Serve over chicken, fish, or vegetables.

Yield: 3 servings

Calories per serving: 61
Calcium: 180 mg
Fat: 0 g
Sodium: 71 mg

Greek Yogurt
Salad Dressing

1	cup low-fat plain yogurt
1	tablespoon buttermilk
½	teaspoon prepared mustard
1	teaspoon olive oil
2	tablespoons lemon juice
2	tablespoons chopped fresh dill

Combine all ingredients.

Yield: 11 servings (2 tablespoons each)

Calories per serving: 19
Calcium: 46 mg
Fat: 1 g
Sodium: 20 mg

Tzadziki Dip

1   cup nonfat plain yogurt
1   small cucumber, grated or minced
1   clove garlic, minced
1   tablespoon olive oil
½   teaspoon vinegar
½   teaspoon lemon juice
1   teaspoon dried dill weed
½   teaspoon dried oregano
1   tablespoon Mock Sour Cream
      (recipe follows), or nonfat sour cream
      pepper to taste

Mix all ingredients well. Serve with toasted pita-bread slices.

Yield: 15 servings (2 tablespoons each)

Calories per serving: 20
Calcium: 35 mg
Fat: 1 g
Sodium: 15 mg

Mock Sour Cream

    1   cup low-fat (1 percent) cottage
          cheese
    2   tablespoons skim milk
    1   tablespoon lemon juice

Place all ingredients in blender or food processor and combine at high speed until thoroughly mixed—at least 1 minute.

Yield: 8 servings (2 teaspoons each)

Snacks and
Desserts

Fruit and Cheese Munchies

1½	ounces low-fat Monterey Jack, mild Cheddar, or Muenster cheese, cut into 8 ½-inch cubes
8	½-inch chunks fresh fruit, such as apple, banana, pincapple, peach, melon

Alternately skewer cheese cubes and fruit chunks on toothpicks.

Yield: 1 serving

Calories per serving: 184
Calcium: 320 mg
Fat: 7 g
Sodium: 136 mg

Holiday Cheese Ring

1	pound reduced-fat sharp Cheddar cheese
1	small onion
1	clove garlic, pressed
¾	cup reduced-fat mayonnaise
½	cup chopped pecans
½	teaspoon Tabasco
1	12-ounce jar strawberry preserves
1	8½-ounce box reduced-fat Triscuits

Grate Cheddar cheese and small onion. Combine with pressed garlic clove, mayonnaise, chopped pecans, and Tabasco. Shape into ring. Serve with strawberry preserves in center of ring, and Triscuits. (Analysis below does not include Triscuits.)

Yield: 20 servings

Calories per serving: 169
Calcium: 169 mg
Fat: 5 g
Sodium: 187 mg

Chocolate Orange Parfaits

2 cups skim milk
1 package sugar-free instant chocolate pudding
½ cup nonfat dry milk powder
¾ teaspoon grated orange peel + more as optional topping
1 cup evaporated skim milk, chilled

In a large bowl, place skim milk, chocolate pudding mix, nonfat dry milk, and orange peel. Mix at low speed until just blended, 1–2 minutes. With a separate chilled bowl and beaters, beat evaporated skim milk until soft peaks form, and fold into thickened pudding. Spoon into dessert glasses. Sprinkle top of each serving with a small amount of grated orange peel if desired.

Yield: 7 servings (½ cup each)

Calories per serving: 115
Calcium: 300 mg
Fat: 2 g
Sodium: 325 mg

Chocolate Pudding

4	cups skim milk
4	tablespoons unsweetened cocoa powder
5	tablespoons cornstarch
4	tablespoons sugar

Combine all ingredients in a blender. Blend until smooth. Pour into a small saucepan over medium-high heat, stirring constantly. Cook, continuing to stir, until it comes to a boil. Remove from heat and pour into a bowl or individual cups. Refrigerate until cold. Serve cold.

Yield: 8 servings (½ cup each)

Calories per serving: 87
Calcium: 155 mg
Fat: 1 g
Sodium: 64 mg

Molasses Cookies

5	egg whites
⅓	cup molasses
⅛	cup apple juice
½	cup canola oil
2	cups sugar
1½	cups all-purpose flour
2½	cups old-fashioned rolled oats
1⅙	cups oat bran
2	teaspoons cinnamon
¾	teaspoon dry ginger
1½	teaspoons baking soda
¼	teaspoon salt
⅛	teaspoon ground cloves

Preheat oven to 350°F. Using a hand mixer, mix egg whites, molasses, apple juice, and oil. In a large bowl, mix together 1 cup of the sugar, the flour, oatmeal, oat bran, cinnamon, ginger, baking soda, salt, and cloves. Combine the wet and dry ingredients together on low speed until blended and moist. Refrigerate batter for 1 hour. Use a 2-ounce scoop to measure cookies. Shape each cookie into a ball, roll it in the reserved cup of sugar, then press down with a rolling pin or jar on a greased baking sheet. Bake cookies for 8 minutes.

Yield: 36 servings (1 cookie per serving)

Calories per serving: 96
Calcium: 40 mg
Fat: 3 g
Sodium: 58 mg

Fudge Pudding Cake

1¼	cups sugar
1	cup all-purpose flour (unsifted)
½	cup unsweetened cocoa powder
2	teaspoons low-sodium baking powder
2	cups skim milk
2	tablespoons reduced-calorie margarine, melted
½	teaspoon pure vanilla extract nonstick spray

Preheat oven to 350°F. In a large bowl, combine ¾ cup of the sugar, the flour, ¼ cup of the cocoa, and the baking powder. With a wooden spoon stir in ½ cup of the milk, the margarine, and the vanilla extract. Spray an 8-inch square baking pan with nonstick spray and spread batter into pan. Sprinkle remaining ½ cup sugar and ¼ cup cocoa over the batter. Pour remaining 1½ cups milk over all. Bake until a knife inserted in the center comes out clean, 30–35 minutes. Let cool on a rack to room temperature before serving.

Yield: 8 servings

Calories per serving: 206 Fat: 2 g
Calcium: 130 mg Sodium: 65 mg

Note: For an added boost of calcium, serve with ½ cup fat-free ice cream. This would add approximately 88 mg of calcium.

Chocolate Cheesecake

3¾	cups low-fat plain or vanilla yogurt drained to 1½ cups
	nonstick spray
2	tablespoons graham-cracker crumbs
1	cup low-fat (1-percent) cottage cheese
1	cup sugar
½	cup unsweetened cocoa powder
¼	cup all-purpose flour
1	teaspoon instant coffee
1	egg
1	egg yolk

Place a paper coffee filter inside a plastic sieve, position sieve over a bowl, and pour yogurt into filter. Allow yogurt to drain overnight in refrigerator. Preheat oven to 300°F. Spray 8-inch springform or cake pan with nonstick spray and dust with crumbs. In food processor or blender, process cottage cheese until smooth; add yogurt, sugar, cocoa, flour, and instant coffee; process until smooth. Add egg and egg yolk; process just until incorporated. Pour batter into pan and bake for 45 minutes, or until set. Refrigerate cheesecake overnight.

Yield: 12 servings

Calories per serving: 161
Calcium: 151 mg
Fat: 3 g
Sodium: 129 mg

Fruit and Yogurt Pie

6	ounces graham-cracker crumbs
½	cup apple juice (or less)
	nonstick spray
2	cups melon cubes
2	tablespoons plain gelatin
½	cup water
2	cups cottage cheese
2	cups low-fat plain yogurt
1	cup sugar
1	teaspoon vanilla extract
	pinch of nutmeg

Put graham-cracker crumbs in blender and blend in apple juice (just enough to moisten crumbs—don't use the full ½ cup). Spray 9-by-9-inch pan with non-stick spray and push crumbs in. Put melon cubes in pan. Sprinkle gelatin over ½ cup of water in small saucepan. Let soften, then gently heat until gelatin dissolves; make sure you *do not* bring to a boil. Set aside. In blender, mix cottage cheese, yogurt, sugar, vanilla, and nutmeg and blend well. Add gelatin while it's still warm and not set. If gelatin is hard, put over low heat just long enough to melt it. Pour blended mix over fruit and chill at least 3 hours.

Yield: 16 servings

Calories per serving: 146
Calcium: 77 mg
Fat: 2 g
Sodium: 203 mg

Trifle

A dessert made from custard, cake, and fresh fruit. The cake portion of the recipe makes twice as much as you'll need for one trifle, so freeze half of it for another time.

Custard:

4	eggs
2	egg whites
¼	cup all-purpose flour
1½	cups sugar
8	cups skim milk
½	vanilla bean, or 1 tablespoon vanilla extract

Cake:

	nonstick spray
1¼	cups all-purpose flour, sifted, + more for dusting
1	egg
1	egg white
6	tablespoons skim milk, warmed
¾	cup sugar
1¼	teaspoons baking powder
	pinch of salt

Fresh Fruit:

8	cups peeled and diced fruit in season, such as mangoes, bananas, strawberries, and kiwis, plus more for optional topping

Combine eggs, egg whites, flour, and sugar in saucepan and whisk until smooth. Add milk and vanilla bean (or extract). Stir constantly over medium-high heat until custard begins to thicken (be careful not to let eggs cook). Remove from heat, strain if not smooth, pour into a shallow pan, and cool in the refrigerator.

Preheat oven to 375°F. Spray an 8-inch cake pan with nonstick spray and dust with flour. Combine and whisk egg, egg white, and warm milk in a bowl. Add sugar and fold in sifted flour, baking powder, and salt. Pour into prepared baking pan and bake for about 15 minutes, or until top of cake is brown and a toothpick inserted into center comes out dry. Let cake cool and cut in half. Wrap one half in aluminum foil and freeze. Cut the other half into ½-inch squares.

To assemble: In a large bowl, put cake on bottom and fruit on top of it, and pour custard over all. You can decorate the top with more fresh fruit.

Yield: 16 servings

Calories per serving: 183
Calcium: 143 mg
Fat: 2 g
Sodium: 95 mg

Chapter Ten

Strategies for Diet Survival Away from Home

E ating out no longer means taking a vacation from healthy eating. Supermarkets and restaurants are catching up with the desire of people to eat more nutritious food from a variety of ethnic traditions. More menus feature offerings that are low in fat and salt. Fortunately for calcium-conscious diners, dairy foods are such a staple of most diets that you can find them at virtually any food outlet in the world. Restaurants are responding to the public's desire for healthier foods by offering low-fat or skim milk and other low-fat dairy fare, making it easier than ever to eat well when away from home. Like anything else well done, eating well-balanced, high-calcium meals away from home requires a little planning, but not a lot.

Dining Out

Office executives, vacationing families, and retirees on the road need to think ahead about where they may obtain their calcium when dining out is on the day's agenda. A beginning strategy is to obtain calcium from dairy sources such as low-fat milk and yogurt at the easiest meals or times available. For example, when possible, grab a high-calcium breakfast before leaving your fully stocked cupboard at home. This eliminates having to shop around for dairy products and assures you a good start on obtaining your daily calcium needs. When that's impossible, consider the easiest meals at which to order low-fat milk or yogurt at restaurants. Continental breakfasts offered at many motels often include milk and yogurt on the menu. Most luncheon establishments, where sandwiches and salads are served, offer a variety of dairy choices to their customers. Grabbing a high-calcium snack such as a yogurt or half-pint of milk, available in most snack bars and convenience stores, can also help fill your daily calcium quota.

Another strategy is to enlist your wait staff in helping you achieve your calcium goals. Depending on the type of restaurant, the staff can be very knowledgeable and informative about menu items and ingredients found in combination dishes. Often such information is not printed on the menu and must be solicited: ask your wait staff if milk or yogurt is available.

If you are not satisfied that you have met your dietary goal of high calcium intake, use a different strategy—look at the menu and discuss with your wait staff menu items and combination dishes that supply generous amounts of calcium. Choose items that contain dairy products such as cheese. Try to choose lower-fat alternatives whenever possible. A grilled-chicken sandwich with Swiss cheese and no mayonnaise would be a relatively low-fat, high-calcium choice. Meatless dishes that contain cheese, such as vegetarian pizza or meatless lasagna, are other smart choices. A baked potato topped with Cheddar cheese is another. Remember that such dairy products as creamy salad dressings, sour cream, mayonnaise, and butter contain relatively no calcium and are loaded with saturated-fat grams. Ask to have these on the side or left off entirely.

Just as you can ask the wait staff to modify dishes to keep the fat grams low, you can ask to have low-fat dairy products added to orders. Ask for Parmesan cheese to sprinkle on pasta, cottage cheese to add to salad, plain yogurt to spoon on potatoes, and a slice of cheese to top a lean-meat sandwich. This strategy works well when there is a large menu and an accommodating chef.

In choosing a dessert, select frozen yogurt or ice cream to boost your calcium consumption. If these choices are not available at the restaurant where you are dining, consider moving on to a yogurt shop or ice-cream shop. It will add some variety to the evening as well as a calcium boost.

The restaurant you choose will determine the variety and availability of high-calcium choices. As you identify establishments that have options to meet your dietary needs, frequent them whenever possible. Consider the menu size and type. Usually a larger menu offers a greater variety of choices, substitutions, and flexibility in preparation. A set menu, where you have identified high-calcium choices, may be a safer bet than a rotating menu. Smaller establishments, however, will often accommodate special requests.

Another strategy is to choose ethnic restaurants that offer many high-calcium choices (see the list on page 152). Italian and Mexican menus contain a rich variety of dishes made with cheese. Be aware that a lot of high-calcium choices are also loaded with fat, especially saturated fat. If your entrée is high-fat, choose low-fat side dishes to accompany it. Although Chinese restaurants offer few if any entrées featuring dairy products, many Chinese dishes contain tofu, a good, relatively low-fat calcium source. Bok choy is another popular Asian food rich in calcium. Read the menu, or ask your wait staff to recommend dishes rich in tofu.

High-Calcium Menu Choices at Restaurants

American

New England clam chowder

Scalloped potatoes

Cheese-and-vegetable omelet

Quiche

Broccoli-and-Swiss-cheese soup

Cheese fondue

French onion soup with Swiss cheese

Chef's salad with cheese

Italian

Vegetable pizza

Meatless lasagna

Cheese ravioli

Manicotti

Cheese-stuffed shells

Fettuccine Alfredo

Mexican

Cheese enchilada

Taco

Quesadilla

Bean-and-cheese burrito

Nachos with cheese

Greek

Spanakopita

Moussaka

Salad with feta cheese

Fast-Food Restaurants

It's the rare traveler who can navigate the wearying rigors of the road without occasionally veering into the drive-through lane of at least one of the highways' ubiquitous fast-food restaurants. The good news is it is as simple as barking "One Big Mac!" to consume 250 milligrams of calcium. The bad news is you'll be gulping down 26 grams of fat, along with 930 milligrams of sodium and 510 calories.

Fast-food meals are not recommended on a daily basis for people who are on low-fat or low-sodium diets for medical reasons. Since occasionally dining at a fast-food restaurant may be unavoidable, be selective in your choices. Some offerings are less fatty and salty than others (see table on pages 160–61).

Most fast-food outlets now serve low-fat milk and frozen dairy products that are rich in calcium and relatively low in fat and sodium. These thirst-quenching treats, a pleasant diversion for children on long trips, are also superior choices to carbonated beverages, which may be high in phosphorus. Phosphorus, you'll remember, may thwart your attempts to consume sufficient calcium by inhibiting absorption of the mineral.

If you (or your children) dislike plain milk or are tempted by soda at restaurants, order chocolate milk or a low-fat milk shake as a compromise. Chocolate milk contains almost as much calcium as skim milk (280 milligrams per cup versus 300). Milk shakes contain even more, and some fast-food restaurants now offer low-fat versions that contain fewer calories.

On the Road

The best source for calcium-rich foods away from home is the same as the best source at home—the supermarket.

Just as most interstate-highway exits boast a flock of fast-food restaurants, many also lead to nearby shopping centers, which invariably house supermarkets. As discussed in chapter eight, supermarkets have responded to customers' interest in healthier foods. They have also responded to the challenge from fast-food chains, by selling meals-to-go and single servings of most fresh foods.

The most obvious food-to-go choices include fruit or single-serving yogurts and milk. But most supermarkets feature extensive delicatessens and bakeries that prepare sandwiches and salads to go; some are already boxed or wrapped. A turkey-and-Swiss-cheese sandwich is just one selection you can probably find here that offers calcium and other nutrients. A number of grocery stores even stock their own salad bars. Here you can build up a meal capitalizing on the vegetables and dairy products such as cheese. Grab a bagel, order an ounce of your favorite cheese from the deli, select a piece of fruit, and you've got a meal almost as quick as the drive-through. A cooler full of cold, single-serving juice bottles usually stands near the deli section to complete your nutritious fast-food shopping.

In the Air

When you are flying to your destination, take advantage of the airlines' offer to provide special meals for customers. Call the airline well in advance of your scheduled flight (at least 24 hours ahead) and request the low-fat meal. You can also request a low-sodium meal if desired. Select low-fat or skim milk with your meal or during the beverage service. Carry with you on the plane portable items such as breakfast bars or low-fat yogurt. You can buy milk, yogurt, ice cream, or frozen yogurt from vendors inside airport terminals.

At Your Destination

Once you arrive at your vacation or business destination, there are several ways you can ensure you don't take a vacation from calcium. Try to choose accommodations with some food facilities, such as a motel room with a small refrigerator, to increase your dining options and cut your food costs. Ask the proprietor or other people who live in the area where you can find good supermarkets and restaurants as well as specialty-food stores. Again, if you can eat breakfast at home, capitalize on the opportunity to drink milk or calcium-fortified orange juice or eat yogurt before going off on a trip.

Sampling local culinary specialties is one of the great joys of travel. If you're on Cape Cod, for instance, try the local New England clam chowder· if you discover a wonderful local bakery, see if cheese Danish is among the offerings. You can experience local ambience and boost your calcium intake by carefully perusing menus.

If you're staying at a condominium or cottage with a well-equipped kitchen, bring a few simple ingredients and cooking utensils so you can prepare meals there. Stock up on milk, yogurt, cheese, and other calcium-rich foods. One attribute of these calcium-rich foods vacationers will appreciate is that they require virtually no elaborate preparation—you can get a generous serving of calcium by downing a glass of milk, instant breakfast, container of fruit yogurt, frozen-yogurt bar, or one-ounce chunk of cheese. One diet strategy for traveling is to make high-calcium breakfasts, lunches, and snacks a high priority so that you can indulge yourself in low-fat, delicious dinners out at restaurants in the evening.

A big part of the pleasure of vacationing is dining out. On business trips, there may be no alternative to eating in restaurants. Fortunately, more and more restaurants offer special heart-healthy entrées and dairy products. Even those that don't, probably offer seafood and a salad bar. It may be more difficult to find high-calcium menu choices at extravagant restaurants. Using some of the strategies for obtaining high-calcium foods at restaurants suggested earlier will help you here, too.

Take time to enjoy the outdoors. For a change, try planning a picnic instead of making a restaurant date. See the table on page 159 for high-calcium picnic ideas.

You should also take time to do some weight-bearing exercise when you travel, to aid your digestion and continue to maintain your body's efficiency in absorbing calcium. A simple walk will do the job. Stop at rest areas, open up your cooler full of calcium-rich foods and drinks, and make time for walking or other weight-bearing exercise.

Packing Snacks

Supplement your meals away from home with high-calcium snacks. Either pack your own in a cooler or grab a yogurt or milk at a convenience store or supermarket.

If there is a refrigerator in your office, bring dairy foods to work for snacks, such as single-serving containers of yogurt and pudding cups.

It is important to keep perishable foods such as dairy products in well-insulated, ice-packed coolers, so that they do not spoil. Plastic, refreezable ice packs are handy, less messy ways to keep a cooler interior cold. Keep the cooler out of the sun, and open it as infrequently as possible. If your car is air-conditioned, keep the cooler in the back seat. Remember, milk products stored in temperatures above 42 degrees Fahrenheit for two hours or longer may spoil.

Milk, cheese, and fruit yogurt travel well in coolers. Buy milk containers with caps, and yogurt with resealable tops, and carry plastic sandwich bags for the cheese, so that these items will be stored in airtight containers after opening.

Remember, it is as easy to pack single containers of chocolate milk as it is to pack cans of soda; if you develop the habit, you'll have calcium-rich drinks available when you get thirsty away from home. You can also pack calcium-fortified fruit juice, which contains about the same amount of calcium as milk. Look for brands that have screw-on caps; this makes them easier to store.

If you will be traveling or working where it will be difficult or impossible to refrigerate snacks, remember that in most supermarkets you can also buy milk that requires no refrigeration in sealed, single-serving boxed containers. Thanks to an ultrapasteurization process, this milk can sit on a shelf as long as five months without spoiling. One eight-ounce box contains 300 milligrams of calcium. This milk, which is what most Europeans drink, may be useful to campers or people embarking on hiking or canoeing trips.

Some foods rich in calcium require no refrigeration. Fortified breakfast bars contain 50 milligrams of calcium or more per seving. Other energy bars and health-food bars that contain nonfat dry milk and other nutrients offer handy, healthy alternatives to standard road-trip snacks such as candy or chips because they are packaged in convenient single-serving wrappers.

Some nuts and dried fruits also offer a fair amount of calcium, although they are high in fat and salt. A ½-cup serving of almonds contains 152 milligrams of calcium; ½ cup of Brazil nuts, 130 milligrams. A few dried fruits are another calcium-rich option. A handful of dried dates contains 60 milligrams of calcium, and ½ cup of dried apricots, 44 milligrams. You can even make your own mix at home. The calcium-conscious consumer's best bet among fresh fruit is a simple orange, which serves up more than 50 milligrams of calcium in addition to lots of vitamin C.

Carry Supplements

By now you should know how many daily calcium servings you need. Remember, one serving of dairy products equals one cup of skim milk or its calcium equivalent, 300 milligrams of calcium. If you are concerned that you may not be able to obtain sufficient calcium away from home, bring along a calcium supplement. If you normally take a supplement but left it at home, don't panic. You can find supplements at any pharmacy and antacids that double as calcium supplements at any supermarket. As mentioned in chapter four, make sure your choice does not contain aluminum, which inhibits calcium absorption.

Packing calcium supplements is especially relevant if you are traveling where it is more difficult to obtain dairy products, or know that you will have limited opportunities to select high-calcium meals. See chapter four for information on how to choose a calcium supplement.

Wherever life's journey takes you, you can get enough calcium to prevent osteoporosis or offset its debilitating effects. As this book demonstrates, meeting your dietary calcium needs is easy—and delicious. By eating enough calcium, getting enough exercise, and perhaps taking hormones, you can avoid joining the 25 million Americans who suffer from osteoporosis. If you already are among their number, you can stay healthier and on your feet longer by enjoying a calcium-rich diet.

It is never too early to discover the benefits of calcium.

Enjoy a Calcium-Rich Picnic

Toss out those phosphorus-heavy, calcium-draining soda cans—you can pack plenty of calcium into a picnic lunch with a little imagination. Make sure your cooler is well stocked with ice or ice packs. Here are some ideas:

Food	Calcium content
Cheeese-and-turkey sandwich on calcium-fortified bread	one ounce Swiss = 270 mg two slices bread = 100 mg
Broccoli spears with dip	½ cup = 70 mg
Fruit salad with yogurt topping	½ cup = 150 mg
Health bars fortified with calcium	one bar – about 200 mg
Almonds	¼ cup = 100 mg
Calcium-fortified juice	one cup = 300 mg
Custard pie	one slice = 150 mg

After picnicking, play some baseball or go for a hike to get some weight-bearing exercise, which will make your bones even stronger. And while you're having fun, your skin will be soaking up vitamin D in the sunshine to further aid your body to absorb calcium.

Calcium Content of Some Fast-Food Restaurant Items (Daily Value Calcium = 1,000 mg)

	Calories	Total Fat (g)	Sodium (mg)	Calcium (mg)
McDonald's				
Big Mac	510	26	930	250
McLean Deluxe with cheese	400	16	1,040	250
Egg McMuffin	290	13	730	150
Bacon, Egg & Cheese Biscuit	450	27	1,310	100
Strawberry Low-Fat Frozen Yogurt Sundae	240	1	85	200
16 oz. Vanilla Shake	310	5	170	350
(Serves 1 percent milk.)				
TCBY				
½ cup plain frozen yogurt:				
No sugar added	80	0	35	80
Nonfat	110	0	45	80
Regular	130	3	50	80
(Does not include toppings and sauces!)				
Burger King				
Croissan'wich with Bacon, Egg & Cheese	350	24	790	not available

Double Whopper with Cheese	960	63	1,360	not available
Double Cheeseburger	600	36	1,040	not available

(Serves 2 percent milk.)

Wendy's

Single with Everything	440	23	860	100
Junior Cheeseburger Deluxe	390	20	820	200
Broccoli and Cheese Baked Potato	460	14	440	250
Cheese Baked Potato	560	23	610	300
Frosty Dairy Dessert, 21 oz.	340	10	200	300

(Serves 2 percent milk.)

Resources

American Dietetic Association
216 West Jackson Boulevard, #800
Chicago, IL 60606-6995

Phone (800)-877-1600

National Osteoporosis Foundation
1150 17th Street, NW
Suite 500
Washington, D.C. 20036

Phone (202)-223-2226
Fax (202)-223-2237

A number of useful, inexpensive publications are available from the National Osteoporosis Foundation, including *Boning Up on Osteoporosis* (Item #A106), *Living with Osteoporosis* (Item #A112), and *The Older Person's Guide to Osteoporosis* (Item #A111). Please contact the N.O.F. for current prices and information on ordering.

General Index

Recipe Index

.